PLANT-BASED SECRETS

The Cookbook With Alternative Versions Recipes of Your Family Favorites to New Complete and Delicious Plant-Based Ideas

Botanika Green Way

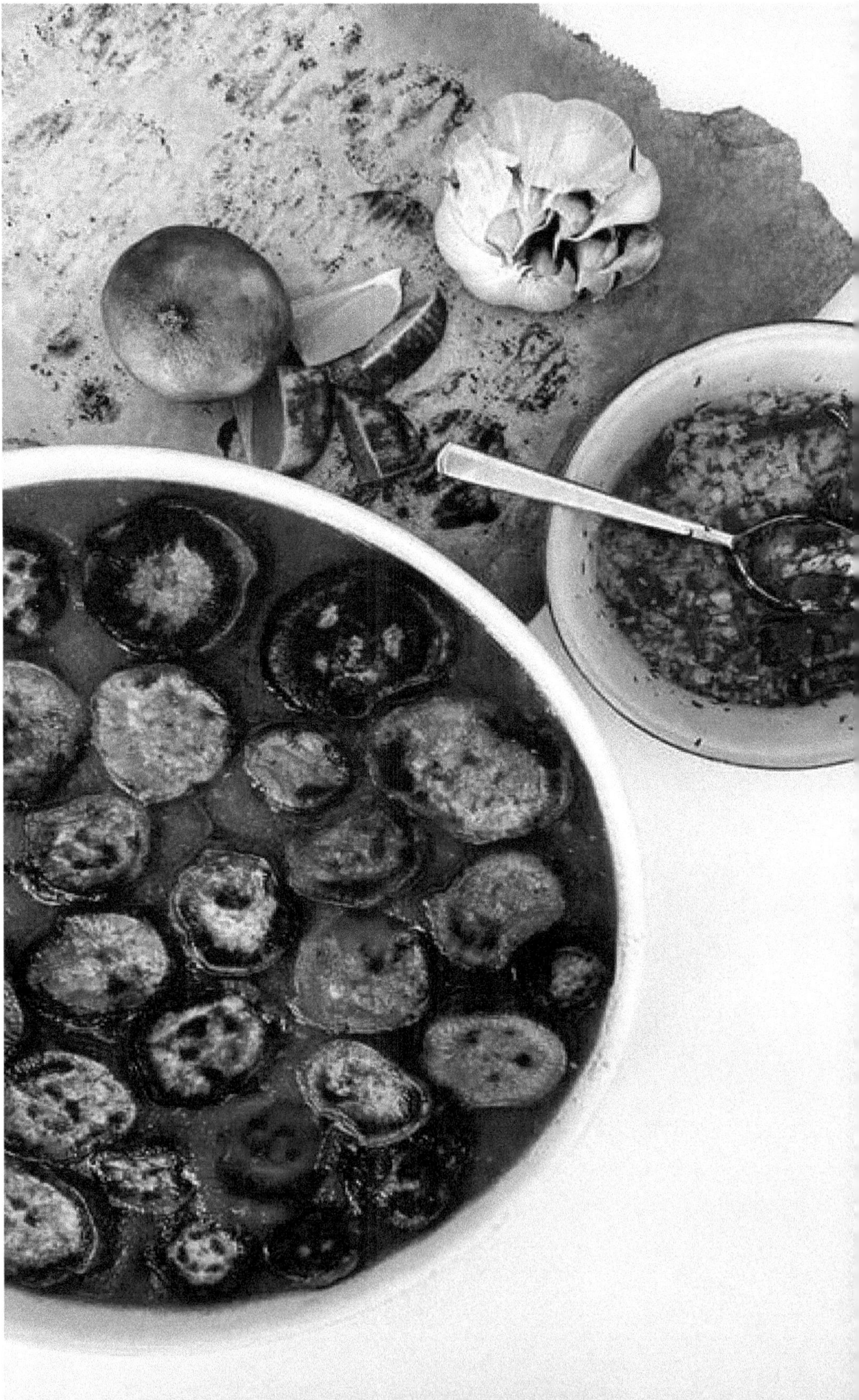

liable for any hardship or damages that may befall them after undertaking the information described herein.

Additionally, the information in the following pages is intended only for informational purposes and should thus be thought of as universal. As befitting its nature, it is presented without assurance regarding its prolonged validity or interim quality. Trademarks that are mentioned are done without written consent and can in no way be considered an endorsement from the trademark holder.

Table of Contents

INTRODUCTION

A plant-based diet is a diet based primarily on whole plant foods. Hence, it excludes animal-sourced foods, hydrogenated oils, refined sugars, and processed foods. A whole food plant-based diet does not consist solely of fruits and vegetables. It includes unprocessed or barely processed oils with healthy fats like extra-virgin olive oil, whole grains, legumes, seeds, and nuts, as well as herbs and spices.

What is the Plant-Based Diet?

The plant-based diet may seem similar to a vegetarian or vegan diet, but it is neither. It's not a diet but a healthy lifestyle. It uses food from plants, and it excludes processed foods like white rice and added sugars, which are allowed in vegan and vegetarian diets.

A plant-based diet is not a diet; it's a healthy way of life

The secret to a healthy diet is simpler than you ever thought! When following a plant-based dietary regimen, you should focus on plant-based foods and avoid animal-sourced food. Whether you are already following a vegan diet or are considering trying this lifestyle, this plant-based, budget-friendly food list makes your grocery shopping easy to manage.

- **VEGETABLES**

Try to include different types of vegetables in your diet from above-ground vegetables to root vegetables, which grow underground.

- **FRUITS**

Choose affordable fruits that are in season. Add frozen fruit to your grocery list since they are just as nutritious as fresh produce. They can be used in smoothies, toppings, compotes, or preserves. On the other hand, dried fruit generally contains a lot of antioxidants, especially polyphenols. It has been proven that eating dried fruits can prevent heart disease and some types of cancer.

- **NUTS & SEEDS**

Nuts and seeds offer different dietary benefits. They do not only ensure essential nutrients but are also offer a variety of flavors. This "ready to eat" food is a perfect snack with dried fruits and trail mix, essential vegan foods to stockpile for an emergency.

- **RICE & GRAINS**

Rice and grains are versatile and easy to incorporate into your diet. Leftovers reheat wonderfully and can be served at any time of the day, turning simple and inexpensive ingredients into a full-fledged meal. You can also make healthy nut butters such as tahini or peanut butter.

- **BEANS & LEGUMES**

Legumes and beans are highly affordable, and there's no end to the variety of tasty dishes you can cook with them. These humble but powerful foods are packed with vitamins, minerals, protein, and dietary fiber. In addition to being super-healthy and versatile, legumes pair very well with other proteins, vegetables, and grains.

- **HEALTHY FATS**

Don't underestimate the importance of quality fats in cooking. Coconut oil, olive oil, and avocado are always good to have on hand.

- **NON-DAIRY PRODUCTS**

Using a plant-based cheese or milk lends flavor, texture, and nutrition to your meals. You can find fantastic products on the market, and this book has many wonderful recipes for feta, vegan ricotta, and plant-based milk.

- **HERBS, SPICES & CONDIMENTS**

A handful of fresh herbs will add that little something extra to your soups, stews, dips, or casseroles. Condiments such as mustard, ketchup, vegan mayonnaise, and plant-based sauces can be used in salads, casseroles, and spreads. Choosing their distinctive flavors to complement vegetables, grains and legumes will help you to make the most of your vegan dishes. Herbs and spices are naturally plant-based, but play it safe and look for a label that says *Vegan-friendly*.

- **BAKING GOODS & CANNED GOODS**

These vegan essentials include all types of flour, baking powder, baking soda, and yeast. Further, cocoa powder, vegan chocolate, and sweeteners are good to have on hand. As for the healthy vegan sweeteners, opt for fresh or dried fruits, agave syrup, maple syrup, and stevia. When it comes to canned goods, stock your pantry with cooking essentials such as tomato, sauerkraut, pickles, low sodium chickpeas and beans, coconut milk, green chilies, pumpkin puree, tomato sauce, low sodium corn, and artichoke hearts. Thus, if you want to make sure you have nutritious, delicious, and quality meals for you and your family, having a vegan pantry is halfway there.

Why You Ought to Reduce Your Intake of Processed and Animal-Based Foods

You have heard over and over that processed food has adverse effects on your health. You might have also been told repeatedly to stay away from foods with lots of preservatives. However, you may have never heard any genuine or concrete facts about why these foods are unsafe. Consequently, let us properly dissect it to help you properly comprehend why you ought to stay away from these offenders.

- **They have massive habit-forming characteristics**

Humans have a predisposition toward being addicted to some specific foods; however, the reality is that the fault is not wholly ours.

Every one of the unhealthy treats we relish now and then triggers a dopamine release. This creates a pleasurable effect in our brain, but the excitement is usually short-lived. The discharged dopamine gradually causes an attachment, and this is the reason some people consistently go back to eat certain unhealthy foods even when they know they're unhealthy and unnecessary. You can get rid of this by avoiding the temptation completely.

- **They are sugar-laden and heavy in glucose-fructose syrup**

Animal-based and processed foods are laden with refined sugars and glucose-fructose syrup, which has almost no nutritional value. An ever-increasing number of studies are affirming what several people presumed from the start: that genetically modified foods bring about inflammatory bowel disease, which consequently makes it increasingly difficult for the body to assimilate essential nutrients. The disadvantages that result from your body being unable to assimilate essential nutrients from consumed foods rightly cannot be overemphasized.

Processed and animal-based food products contain plenteous amounts of refined carbohydrates. Indeed, your body requires carbohydrates to give it energy to function.

In any case, refining carbs dispenses with the fundamental supplements in the way that refining entire grains disposes of the whole grain part. What remains in the wake of refining is what's considered empty carbs or empty calories. These can negatively affect the metabolic system in your body by sharply increasing your blood sugar and insulin levels.

- **They contain lots of synthetic ingredients**

When your body takes in non-natural ingredients, it regards them as of foreign substance and a health threat. It isn't accustomed to identifying synthetic compounds like sucralose or synthesized sugars. Hence, in defense of your health against this foreign "aggressor," your body does what it's programmed to do to safeguard your health: It sets off an immune reaction to tackle this "enemy" compound, which indirectly weakens your body's general disease alertness, making you susceptible to illnesses. The energy expended by your body in triggering your immune system could be better utilized somewhere else.

- **They contain constituent elements that set off a sensation in your body**

A part of processed and animal-based foods contains compounds like glucose-fructose syrup, monosodium glutamate, and specific food dyes that can trigger some addictions. They teach your body to receive a benefit whenever you consume them. Monosodium glutamate, for example, is added to many store-bought baked foods. This additive slowly conditions your palate to relish and crave the taste.

- **This reward-centric arrangement makes you crave it increasingly, which ends up exposing you to the danger of over-consuming calories**

For animal protein, usually, the expression "subpar" is used to allude to plant proteins since they generally have lower levels of essential amino acids as against animal-sourced protein. Nevertheless, what the vast majority don't know is that large amounts of essential amino acids can prove detrimental to your health. Let me break it down further for you.

- **Animal-sourced protein has no fiber**

In their pursuit to consume animal protein, the vast majority wind up dislodging the plant protein that was previously available in their body. Replacing the plant proteins with its animal variant is harmful because, in contrast to plant protein, animal proteins typically are deficient in fiber, phyto-nutrients, and antioxidant properties. Fiber insufficiency is a regular feature across various regions and societies on the planet. In America, for example, according to the National Academy of Medicine, the typical adult takes in roughly 15 grams of dietary fiber daily rather than the recommended daily quantity of 25 to 30 grams. A deficiency in dietary fiber often leads to a heightened risk of breast and colorectal cancers, in addition to constipation, inflammatory bowel disease, and cardiovascular disease.

- **Animal protein brings about an upsurge in phosphorus levels in the body**

Animal protein has significant levels of phosphorus. Our bodies stabilize these plenteous amounts of phosphorus by producing and discharging a hormone known as fibroblast growth factor 23 (FGF23). Studies have shown that this hormone is dangerous to our veins. FGF23 also causes asymmetrical expansion of heart muscles—a determinant for congestive heart failure and even mortality in some advanced cases.

Having discussed the many problems associated with animal protein, it becomes more apt to replace its "high quality" perception with the tag "highly hazardous." In contrast to caffeine, which has a withdrawal effect if it's discontinued abruptly, you can stop taking processed and animal-based foods right away without any withdrawals. Possibly the only thing that you'll give up is the ease of some meals taking little to no time to prepare.

Health Benefits of the Plant-Based Diet

Plant-based eating is one of the healthiest diets in the world. It should include plenty of fresh products, whole grains, legumes, and healthy fats such as seeds and nuts, which are rich in antioxidants, minerals, vitamins, and dietary fiber.

Scientific research has shown that higher use of plant-based foods is connected to a lower risk of death from conditions such as cardiovascular disease, diabetes, hypertension, and obesity. Vegan eating relies heavily on healthy staples, avoiding animal products. Animal products contain much more fat than plant-based foods; it's not a shocker that studies have shown that meat-eaters have nine times the obesity rate of vegans.

This leads us to the next point, one of the greatest benefits of the vegan diet: weight loss. While many people choose to live a vegan life for ethical reasons, the diet itself can help you achieve your weight loss goals. If you're struggling to shift pounds, you may want to consider trying a plant-based diet. How exactly? As a vegan, you will reduce the number of high-calorie foods such as full-fat dairy products, fatty fish, pork, and other cholesterol-containing foods such as eggs. Try replacing such foods with high-fiber and protein-rich alternatives that will keep you fuller longer. The key is focusing on nutrient-dense, clean and natural foods and avoiding empty calories such as sugar, saturated fats, and highly processed foods. Here are a few tricks that help me maintain my weight on the vegan diet. I eat vegetables as a main course; I consume good fats in moderation (good fats such as olive oil do not make you fat); I exercise regularly and cook at home. Plant foods are an excellent source of many nutrients that boost the body's metabolism in many ways. They are easy to digest thanks to their rich content of antioxidants.

- **Reduced Risk of Heart Diseases**

Processed and animal foods are responsible for much heart disease. A whole foods plant-based diet is better at nourishing the body with essential nutrients while improving the heart's function to produce and transport blood to and from the various body parts.

- **Prevents and Heals Diabetes**

Plant-based foods are excellent at reducing high blood sugar. Many studies comparing a vegetarian and vegan diet to a regular meat-filled diet proved that dieting with more plant foods reduced the risk of diabetes by 50 percent.

- **Improved Cognitive Incline**

Fruits and vegetables are excellent for cleansing and boosting metabolism. They release high numbers of plant compounds and antioxidants that slow or prevent cognitive decline. On a plant-based diet, the brain is boosted with sustainable energy, promoting sharp memory, language, thinking, and judgment abilities.

- **Quick Weight Loss**

A high animal food diet is known to drive weight gain. Switching to a plant-based diet helps the body shed fat walls easily, which quickly drives weight loss.

BREAKFAST

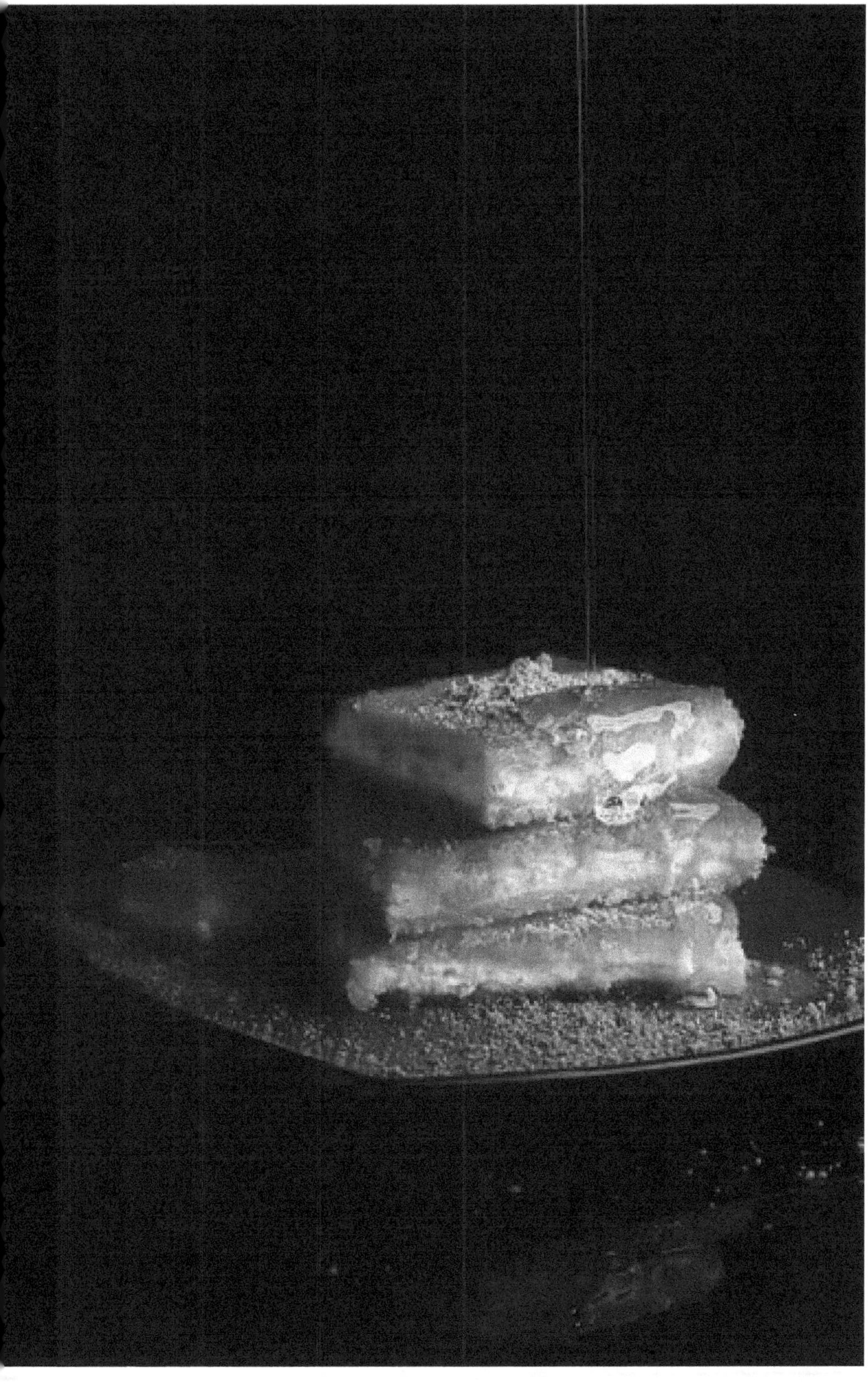

Sweet Kiwi Oatmeal Bars

8 Servings

Preparation Time: 50 minutes

Ingredients

- 2 cups uncooked rolled Oats
- ½ tsp ground Cinnamon
- 1 cup Plant butter, melted
- 4 cups Kiwi, chopped
- ¼ cup Organic cane sugar
- 2 tbsps Cornstarch
- 2 cups All-purpose flour
- 1 ½ cups Pure date sugar
- 1 ½ tsps Baking soda

Directions

- Preheat oven to 380°F. Grease a baking dish.

- In a bowl, mix the oats, flour, date sugar, baking soda, salt, and cinnamon.

- Put in butter and whisk to combine.

- In another bowl, mix the kiwis, cane sugar, and cornstarch until the kiwis are coated.

- Spread 3 cups of oatmeal mixture on a greased baking dish and top with kiwi mixture, and finally put the remaining oatmeal mixture on top.

- Bake for 40 minutes. Allow cooling and slice into bars.

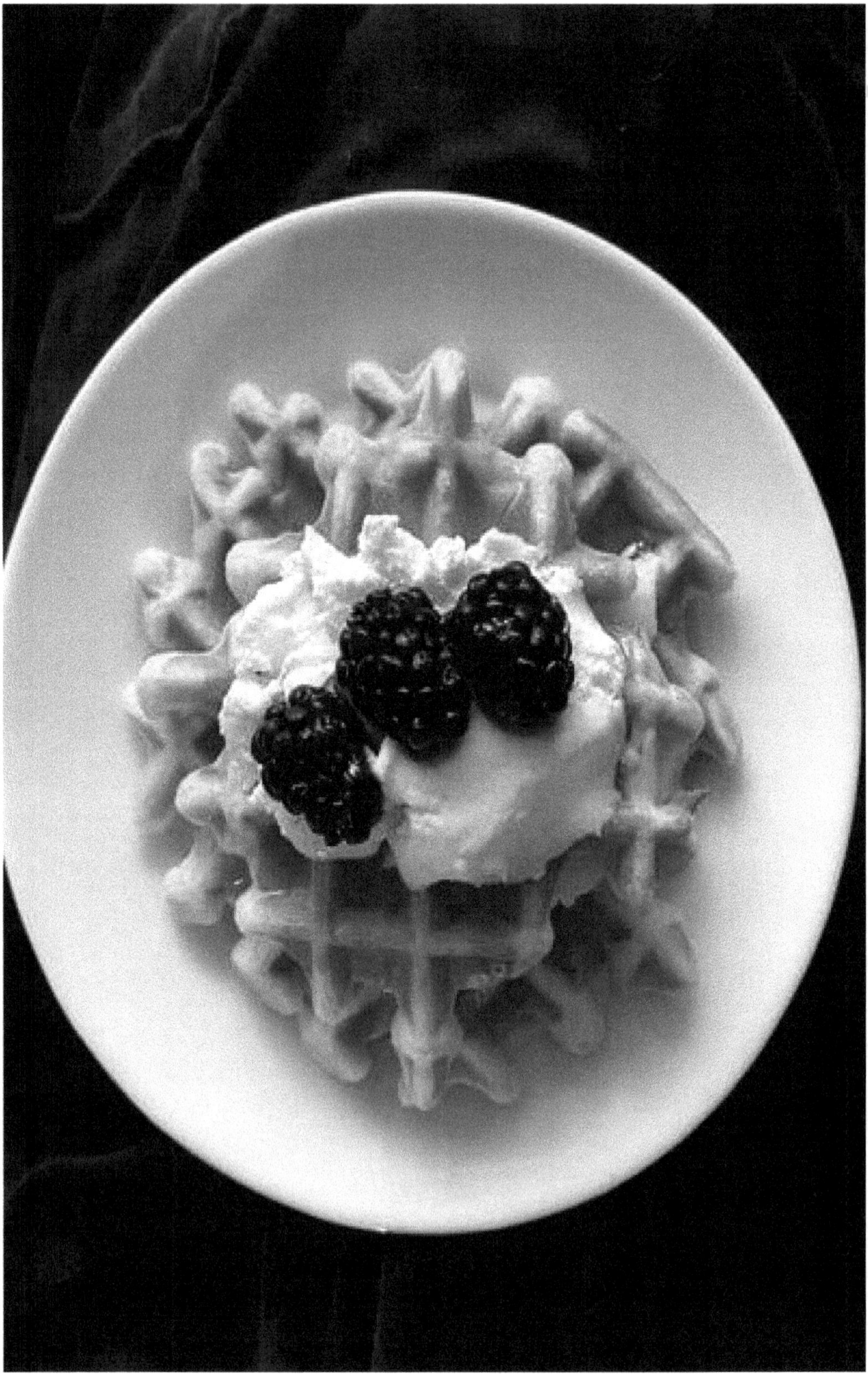

Spicy Apple Pancakes

6 Servings

Preparation Time: 30 minutes

Ingredients

- 2 cups Almond milk
- ½ tsp ground Cinnamon
- ¼ tsp grated Nutmeg
- ¼ tsp ground Allspice
- ½ cup Applesauce
- 1 cup Water
- 1 tbsp Coconut oil
- 1 tsp Apple cider vinegar
- 2 ½ cups Whole-wheat flour
- 2 tbsps Baking powder
- ½ tsp Baking soda
- 1 tsp Sea salt

Directions

- Mix the almond milk and apple cider vinegar in a bowl and set aside.

- In another bowl, mix the flour, baking powder, baking soda, salt, cinnamon, nutmeg, and allspice.

- Transfer the almond mixture to another bowl and beat with the applesauce and water.

- Add in the dry ingredients and stir.

- Melt some coconut oil in a pan over medium heat.

- Pour a ladle of the batter and cook for 5 minutes, flipping once until golden.

- Repeat the process until the batter is exhausted. Serve warm.

Almond & Coconut Granola with Cherries

8 Servings

Preparation Time: 45 minutes

Ingredients

- ½ cup Coconut oil, melted
- ½ cup Maple syrup
- ⅓ cup Whole-wheat flour
- ¼ cup ground Flaxseed
- ½ cup Sunflower seeds
- ½ cup Slivered almonds
- ½ cup shredded Coconut
- ½ cup dried Cherries
- ½ cup dried Apricots, chopped
- 1 tsp Vanilla extract
- 3 tsps Pumpkin pie spice
- 4 cups Rolled oats

Directions

- Preheat oven to 350°F.

- In a bowl, mix the coconut oil, maple syrup, and vanilla.

- Add in the pumpkin pie spice.

- Put oats, flour, flaxseed, sunflower seeds, almonds, and coconut in a baking sheet and toss to combine.

- Coat with the oil mixture. Spread the granola out evenly. Bake for 25 minutes.

- Once ready, break the granola into chunks and stir in the cherries and apricots.

- Bake another 5 minutes. Allow cooling and serve.

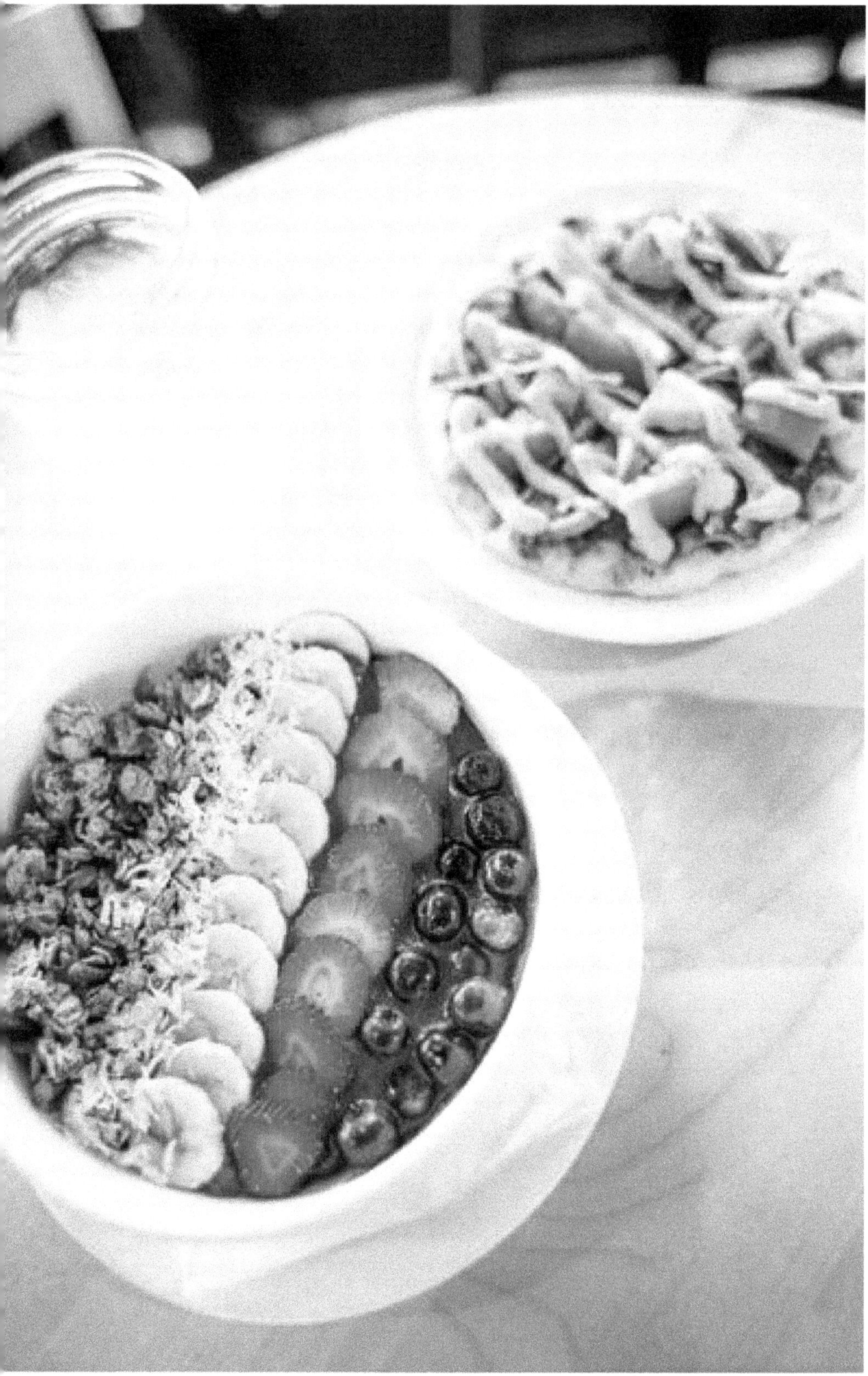

Cinnamon Buckwheat with Almonds

6 Servings

Preparation Time: 20 minutes

Ingredients

- 1 cup Almond milk
- 1 tsp Cinnamon
- ¼ cup chopped Almonds
- 2 tbsps pure Date syrup
- 1 cup Water
- 1 cup Buckwheat groats, rinsed

Directions

- Place almond milk, water, and buckwheat in a pot over medium heat and bring to a boil.

- Lower the heat and simmer covered for 15 minutes. Allow sitting covered for 5 minutes.

- Mix in the cinnamon, almonds, and date syrup. Serve warm.

Maple Banana Oats

6 Servings

Preparation Time: 35 minutes

Ingredients

- 3 cups Water
- 2 Bananas, mashed
- ¼ cup Pumpkin seeds
- 2 tbsps Maple syrup
- A pinch of Salt
- 1 cup steel-cut Oats

Directions

- Bring water to a boil in a pot, add in oats, and lower the heat. Cook for 20-30 minutes.

- Put in the mashed bananas, cook for 3-5 minutes more.

- Stir in maple syrup, pumpkin seeds, and salt. Serve.

Thyme Pumpkin Stir-Fry

4 Servings

Preparation Time: 25 minutes

Ingredients

- 1 cup Pumpkin, shredded
- 2 Garlic cloves, minced
- ½ tsp Dried thyme
- 1 cup chopped Kale
- Salt and Black pepper to taste
- 1 tbsp Olive oil
- ½ Onion, chopped
- 1 Carrot, peeled and chopped

Directions

- Heat the oil in a pan over medium heat. Sauté onion and carrot for 5 minutes.

- Add in the garlic and thyme, cook for 30 seconds until the garlic is fragrant.

- Put in the pumpkin and cook for 10 minutes until tender. Stir in kale, cook for 4 minutes until the kale wilts.

- Season with salt and pepper. Serve hot.

Maple Blueberry Smoothie

6 Servings

Preparation Time: 5 minutes

Ingredients

- 4 cups chopped Arugula
- 4 cups unsweetened Almond milk
- Juice of 2 Limes
- 4 tbsps Maple syrup
- 2 cups frozen Blueberries

Directions

- In a blender, blend the arugula, blueberries, almond milk, lime juice, and maple syrup until smooth. Serve.

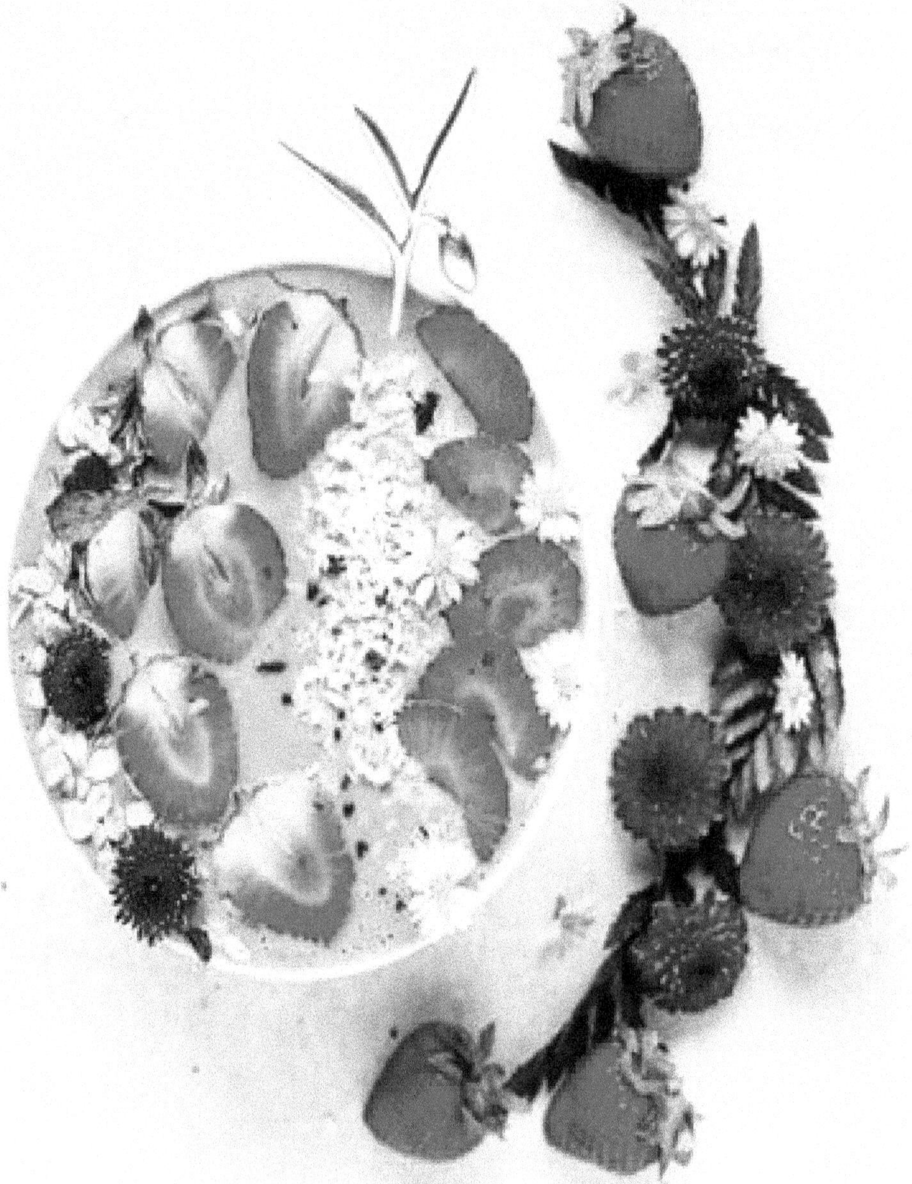

DRINKS

Hibiscus Tea

2 Servings

Preparation Time: 1 minute

Ingredients

- 1 tablespoon of raisins, diced
- 6 Almonds, raw and unsalted
- ½ teaspoon of hibiscus powder
- 2 cups of water

Directions

- Bring the water to a boil in a small saucepan; add in the hibiscus powder and raisins. Give it a good stir, cover, and let simmer for a further two minutes.
- Strain into a teapot and serve with a side helping of almonds.

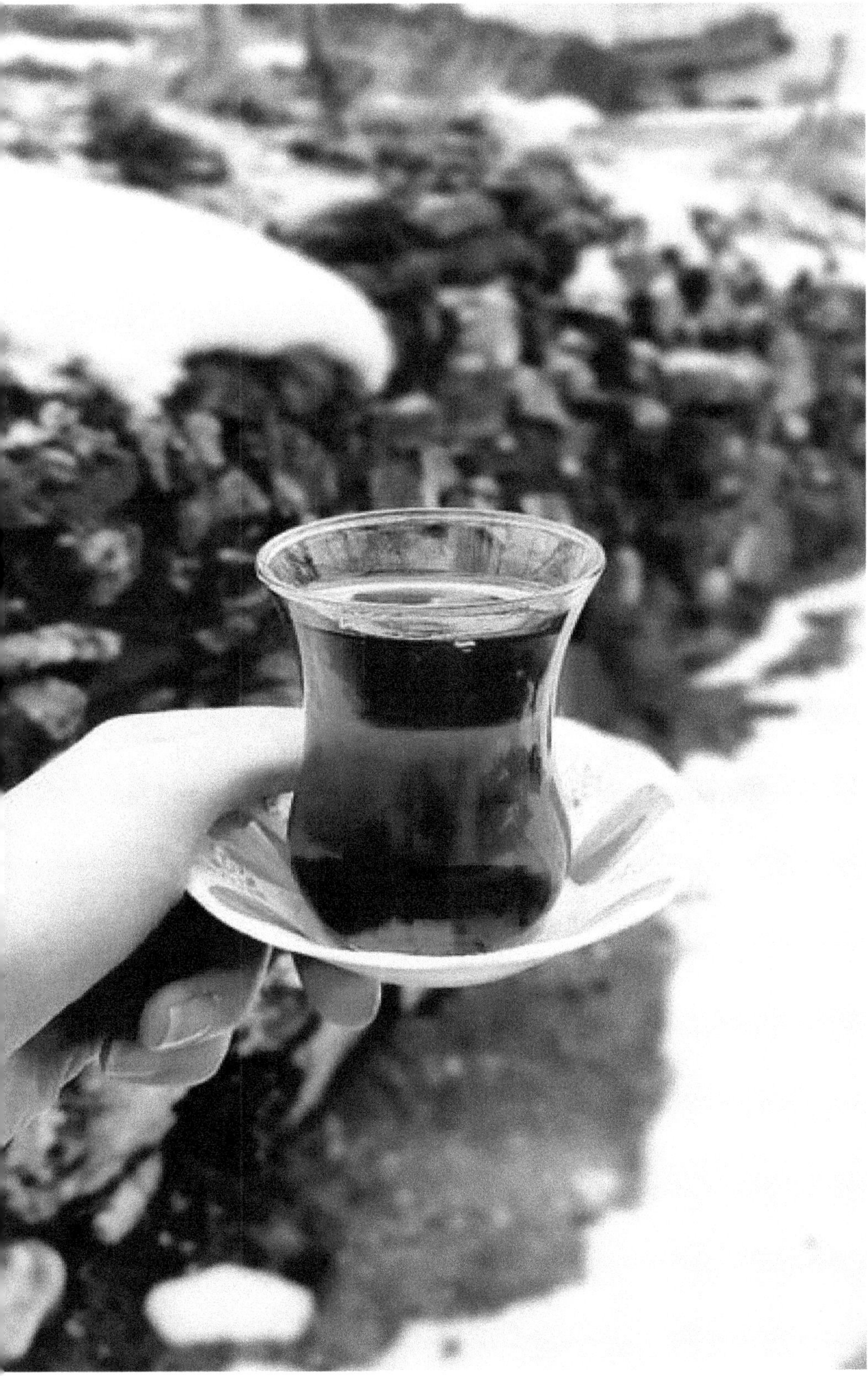

Lemon and Rosemary Iced Tea

4 Servings

Preparation Time: 5 minutes

Ingredients

- 4 cups of water
- 4 earl grey tea bags
- ¼ cup of sugar
- 2 lemons
- 1 sprig of rosemary

Directions

- Peel the two lemons and set the fruit aside.
- In a medium saucepan, over medium heat combine the water, sugar, and lemon peels. Bring this to a boil.
- Remove from the heat and place the rosemary and tea into the mixture. Cover the saucepan and steep for five minutes.
- Add the juice of the two peeled lemons to the mixture, strain, chill, and serve.

Fragrant Spiced Coffee

6 Servings

Preparation Time: 15 minutes

Ingredients

- 4 cinnamon sticks, each about 3 inches long
- 1 1/2 teaspoons of whole cloves
- 1/3 cup of honey
- 2-ounce of chocolate syrup
- 1/2 teaspoon of anise extract
- 6 cups of brewed coffee

Directions

- Pour the coffee into a 4-quarts slow cooker and pour in the remaining ingredients except for cinnamon and stir properly.
- Wrap the whole cloves in cheesecloth and tie its corners with strings.
- Immerse this cheesecloth bag in the liquid present in the slow cooker and cover it with the lid.
- Then plug in the slow cooker and let it cook on the low heat setting for 3 hours or until heated thoroughly.
- When done, discard the cheesecloth bag and serve.

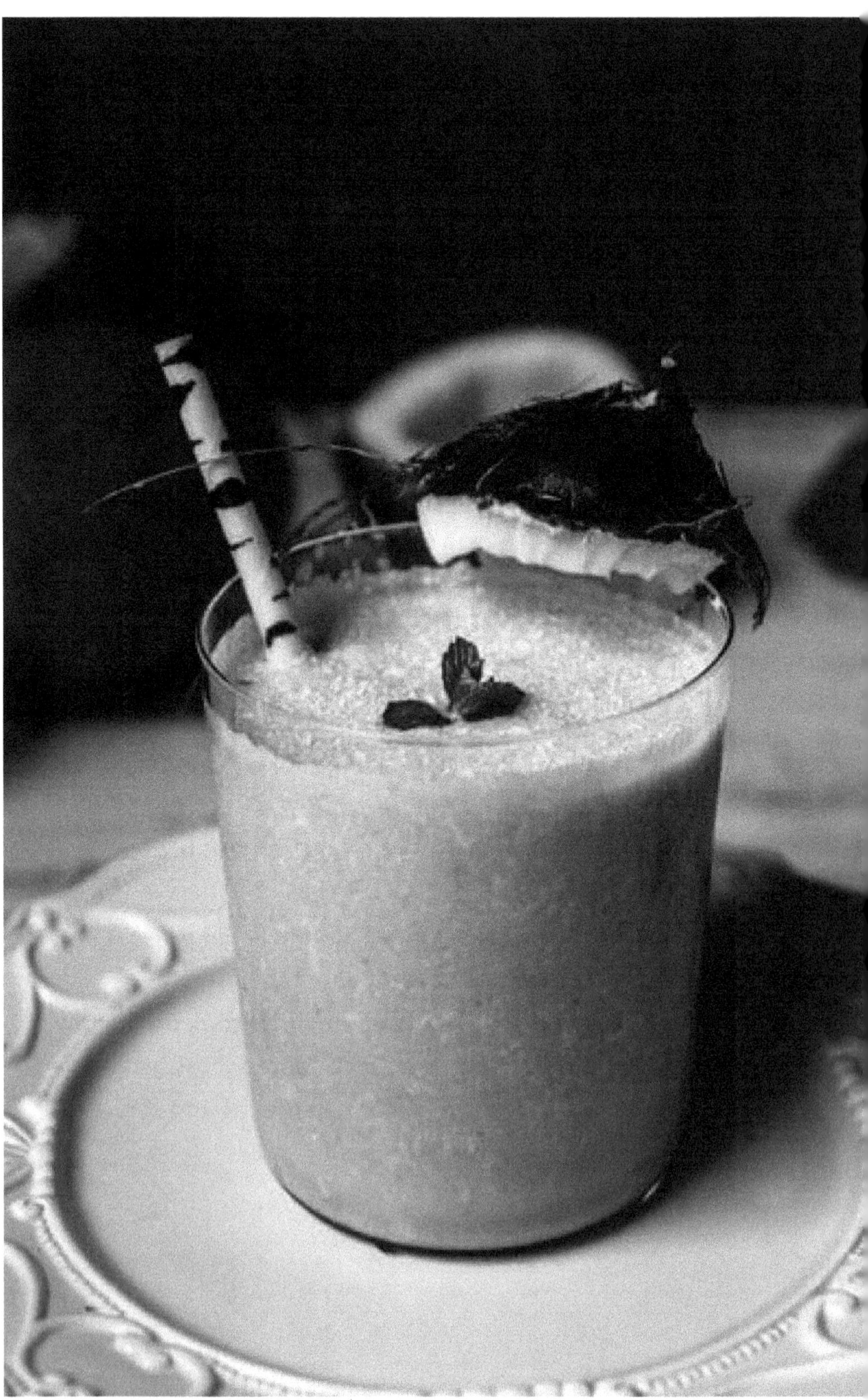

Bracing Coffee Smoothie

1 Serving

Preparation Time: 5 minutes

Ingredients

- 1 banana, sliced and frozen
- ½ cup strong brewed coffee
- ½ cup milk
- ¼ cup rolled oats
- 1 tsp nut butter

Directions

- Mix all the ingredients until smooth.
- Enjoy your morning drink!

LUNCH

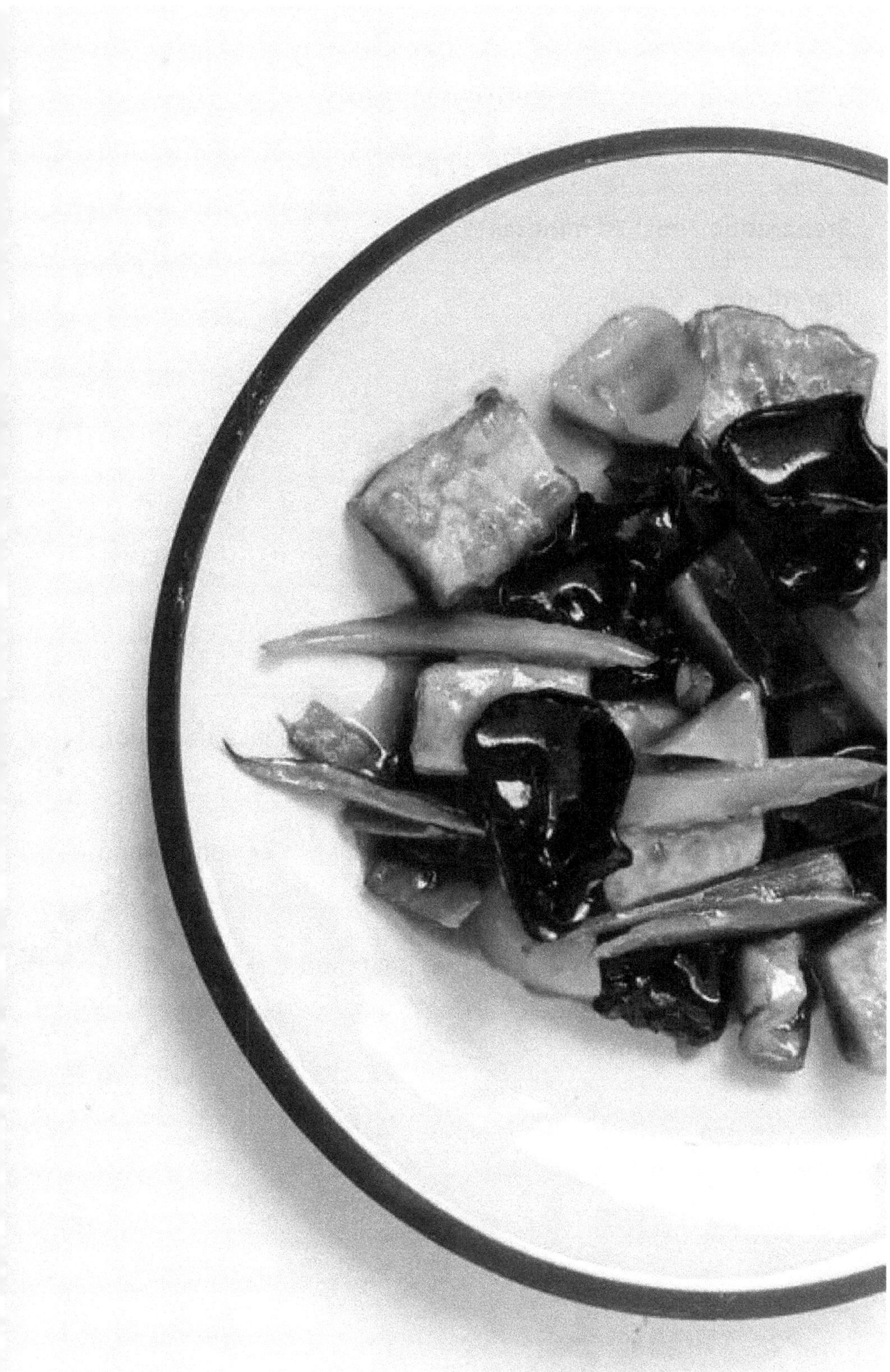

Hot Paprika Lentils

6 Servings

Preparation Time: 20 minutes

Ingredients

- 1 Onion, chopped
- 2 ¼ cups lentils, drained
- 3 garlic cloves, minced
- ½ tsp dried thyme
- 3 tbsps olive oil
- 1 tbsp hot Paprika

Directions

- Heat the oil in a pot over medium heat. Place the onion and garlic and sauté for 3 minutes.

- Add in paprika, salt, pepper, 5 cups water, lentils, and thyme.

- Bring to a boil, lower the heat and simmer for 15 minutes until tender, stirring often.

Chipotle Kidney Bean Chili

6 Servings

Preparation Time: 30 minutes

Ingredients

- 2 tbsps olive oil
- 1 canned chipotle chili, minced
- 1 tsp ground cumin
- ½ tsp dried marjoram
- 1 (15.5-oz) can kidney beans
- Salt and black pepper to taste
- ½ tsp cayenne pepper
- 1 onion, chopped
- 2 garlic cloves, minced
- 1 (16-oz) can tomato sauce
- 1 (4-oz) can green chilies, chopped
- 1 tbsp chili powder

Directions

- Heat the oil in a pot over medium heat.

- Place in onion and garlic and sauté for 3 minutes.

- Put in tomato sauce, green chilies, chili powder, cumin, cayenne pepper, marjoram, salt, and pepper and cook for 5 minutes.

- Stir in kidney beans and 2 cups of water. Bring to a boil, then lower the heat and simmer for 15 minutes, stirring often. Serve immediately.

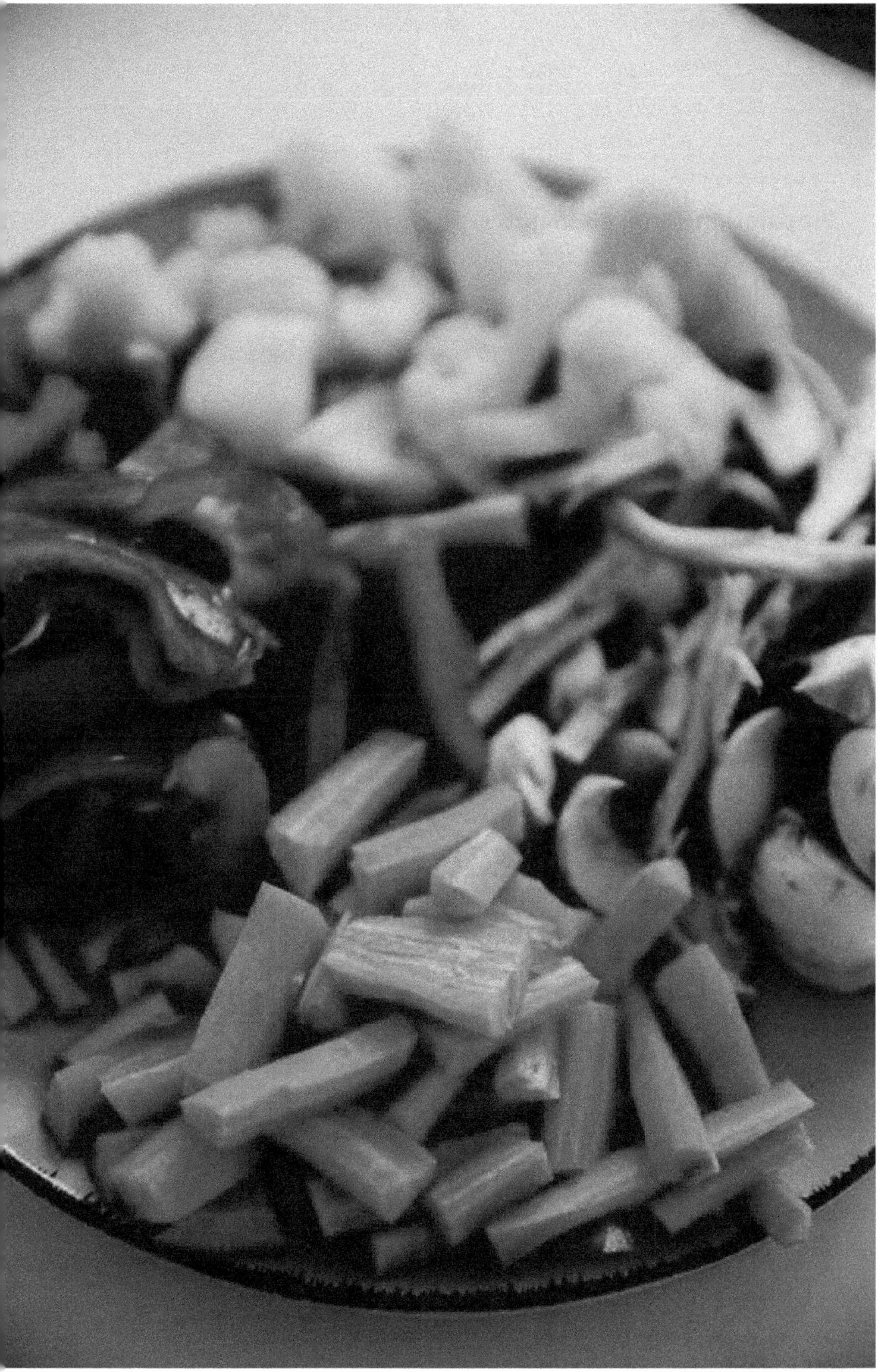

Carrot & Black Bean Chili

6 Servings

Preparation Time: 25 minutes

Ingredients

- 2 tbsps olive oil
- 2 tbsps chili powder
- 1 (28-oz) can diced tomatoes
- 1 (15.5-oz) can black beans
- 3 minced green onions
- 1 onion, finely chopped
- 2 carrots, chopped
- 1 tsp grated fresh ginger
- 1 green bell pepper, chopped

Directions

- Heat the oil in a pot over medium heat. Place in onion, carrot, ginger, bell pepper, and chili powder and sauté for 5 minutes until tender.

- Stir in tomatoes, 2 cups of water, black beans, salt, and pepper.

- Bring to a boil, then lower the heat and simmer for 15 minutes.

- Serve topped with green onions.

Special Butternut Squash Chili

6 Servings

Preparation Time: 60 minutes

Ingredients

- 1 butternut squash, cubed
- 1 (15.5-oz) can garbanzo beans
- 1 cup frozen green peas
- 1 cup corn kernels
- ½ tsp cayenne pepper
- ½ tsp ground allspice
- 2 tbsps olive oil
- 1 onion, chopped
- 3 cups tomato salsa

Directions

- Heat the oil in a saucepan over medium heat.

- Place in onion and squash and cook for 10 minutes until tender.

- Add in tomato salsa, garbanzo beans, green peas, corn, cayenne pepper, allspice, salt, and pepper. Pour in 2 cups of water.

- Bring to a boil, then lower the heat and simmer for 15 minutes. Serve.

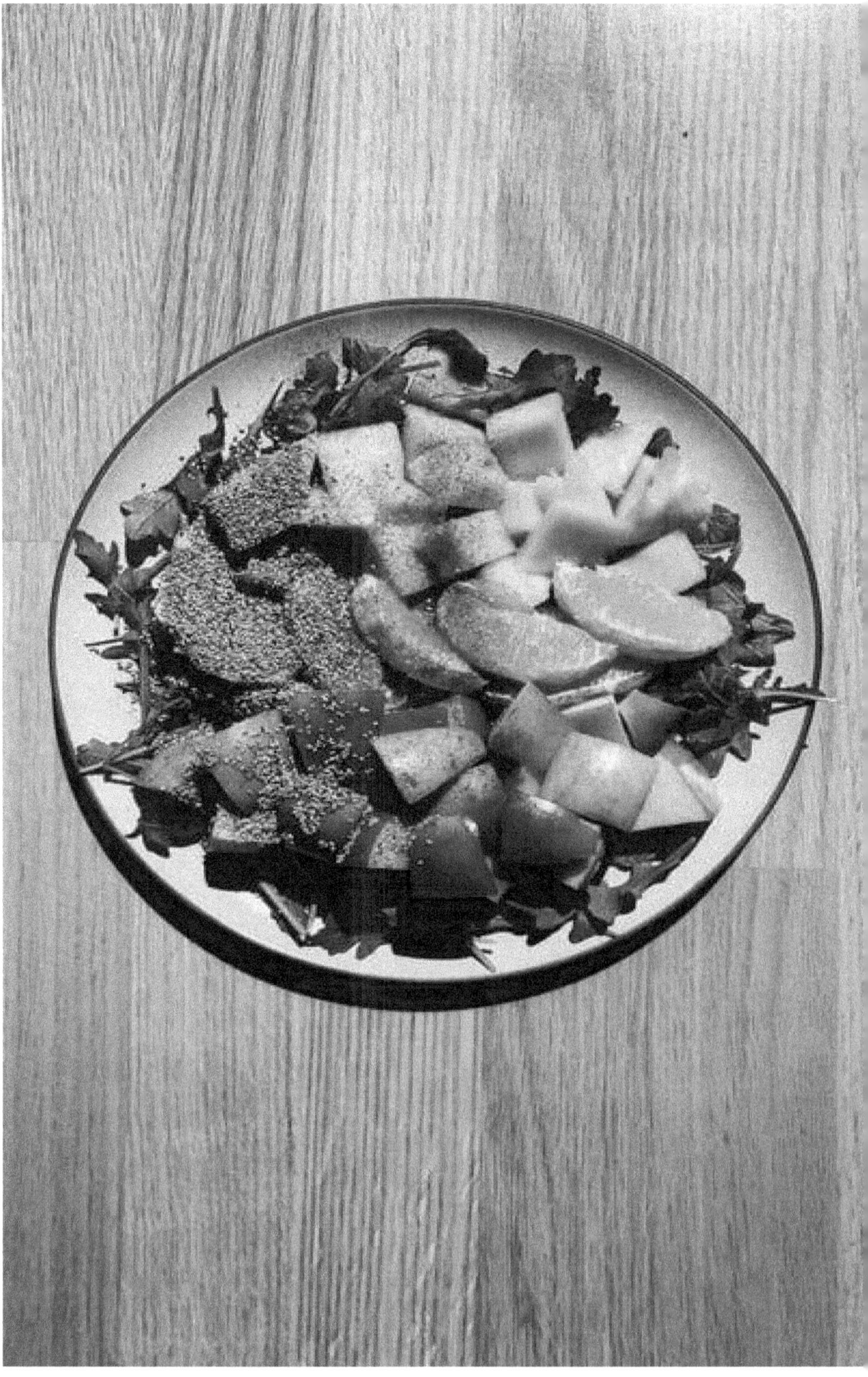

Mediterranean Chickpeas with Vegetables

8 Servings

Preparation Time: 40 minutes

Ingredients

- 3 tbsps olive oil
- 2 parsnips, peeled and chopped
- 8 oz green beans, chopped
- 1 (15.5-oz) can chickpeas, drained
- 1 (14.5-oz) can diced tomatoes
- 1 ½ cups vegetable broth
- 2 tbsps minced cilantro
- 1 tsp fresh lemon juice
- 1 red onion, chopped
- 2 carrots, chopped
- 1 celery stalk, chopped
- 2 garlic cloves, minced
- 1 tsp grated fresh ginger
- 1 tsp ground cumin
- ½ tsp turmeric

Directions

- Heat the oil in a pot over medium heat. Place in onion, carrots, celery, garlic, and ginger. Sauté for 5 minutes.

- Add in cumin, turmeric, parsnips, green beans, chickpeas, tomatoes and juices, and broth.

- Bring to a boil, then lower the heat and sprinkle with salt and pepper. Simmer for 30 minutes.

- Sprinkle with lemon juice and cilantro and serve.

Southern Bean Salad

6 Servings

Preparation Time: 15 minutes

Ingredients

- 1 Tomato, chopped
- 2 Avocados, pitted
- 1 tbsp Lemon juice
- ¼ cup sake
- 1 tsp dried oregano
- Salt to taste
- 2 tbsps Olive oil
- 1 cup leafy greens, chopped
- 1 red bell pepper, chopped
- 1 green bell pepper, chopped
- 1 small red onion, sliced
- 1 (14.5-oz) can black-eyed peas
- 1 (14.5-oz) can black beans
- ¼ cup capers

Directions

- In a bowl, mix the tomato, peppers, onion, black-eyed peas, beans, and capers.

- Put the avocados, lemon juice, sake, olive oil, oregano, and salt in a food processor and blitz until smooth.

- Add the dressing to the bean bowl and toss to combine.

- Transfer to a plate and top with leafy greens to serve.

Hot Coconut Beans with Vegetables

6 Servings

Preparation Time: 18 minutes

Ingredients

- 2 tbsps olive oil
- 1 (13.5-oz) can coconut milk
- 2 (15.5-oz) cans white beans
- 1 (14.5-oz) can diced tomatoes
- 3 cups fresh baby spinach
- Salt and black pepper to taste
- Chopped toasted walnuts
- 1 onion, chopped
- 1 red bell pepper, chopped
- 2 garlic cloves, minced
- 1 tbsp hot powder
- 2 tbsps plant butter

Directions

- Heat the oil in a pot over medium heat.

- Place in onion, garlic, hot powder, and bell pepper and sauté for 5 minutes, stirring occasionally.

- Put in butter and coconut milk and whisk until well mixed

- . Add in white beans, tomatoes, spinach, salt, and pepper and cook for 5 minutes until the spinach wilts.

- Transfer to a platter, garnish with walnuts and serve.

Seitan & Lentil Chili

6 Servings

Preparation Time: 35 minutes

Ingredients

- 2 tbsps olive oil
- 1 tsp ground cumin
- 1 tsp ground allspice
- ½ tsp ground oregano
- ¼ tsp ground cayenne
- Salt and black pepper to taste
- 1 onion, chopped
- 8 oz seitan, chopped
- 1 cup lentils
- 1 (14.5-oz) can diced tomatoes
- 1 tbsp soy sauce
- 1 tbsp chili powder

Directions

- Heat the oil in a pot over medium heat. Place in onion and seitan and cook for 10 minutes.

- Add in lentils, diced tomatoes, 2 cups of water, soy sauce, chili powder, cumin, allspice, sugar, oregano, cayenne pepper, salt, and pepper.

- Bring to a boil, then lower the heat and simmer for 20 minutes.

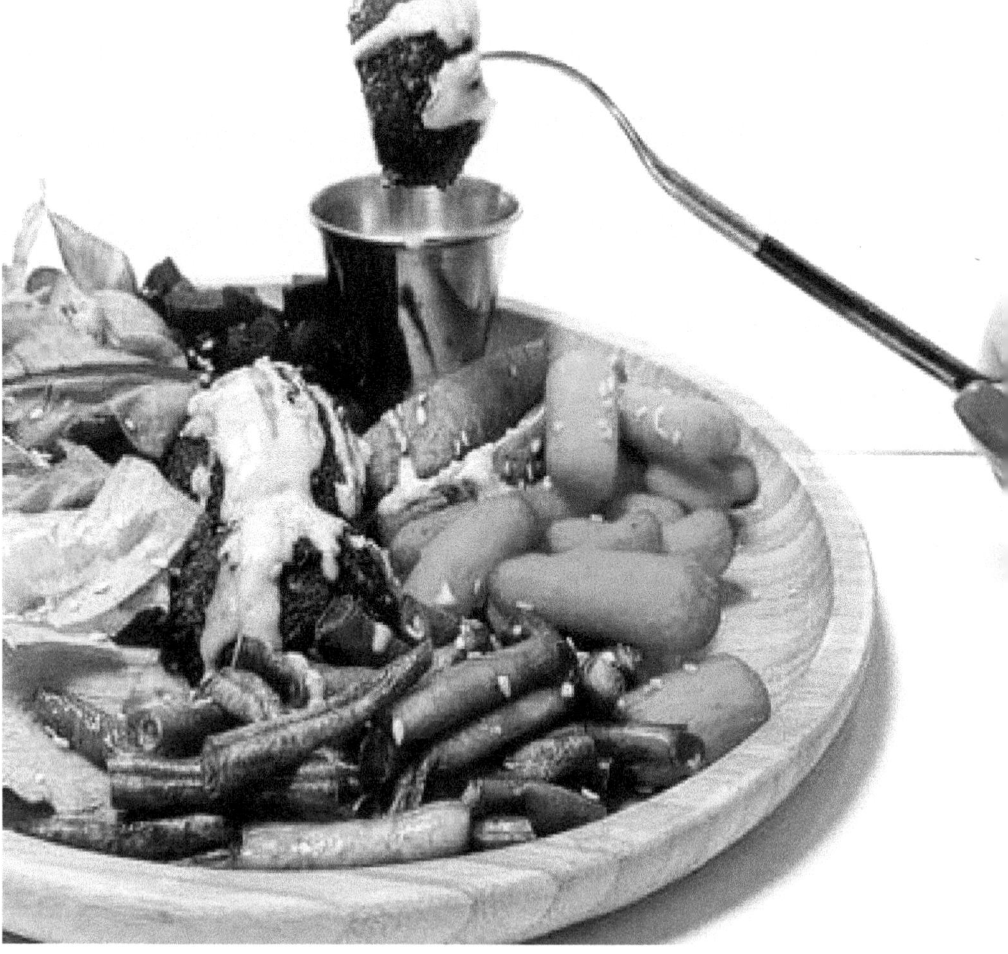

White Salad with Walnut Pesto

6 Servings

Preparation Time: 25 minutes

Ingredients

- 1 lb potatoes, cut into chunks
- ½ cup chopped fresh parsley
- ¼ cup walnut oil
- ¼ cup olive oil
- ¼ cup white wine vinegar
- Salt to taste
- ¼ tsp crushed red pepper
- 3 cups cauliflower florets
- 1 (15.5-oz) can cannellini beans
- ½ cup Kalamata olives, halved
- ½ cup walnuts
- 2 garlic cloves, minced

Directions

- Cook the potatoes for 15 minutes in salted water.

- Add in the cauliflower and cook for another 5 minutes until the veggies are tender. Drain and remove to a bowl.

- Stir in beans, olives, and half of the walnuts.

- In a blender, mix the remaining walnuts, garlic, parsley, walnut oil, olive oil, vinegar, salt, sugar, and red pepper.

- Blitz until well blended. Pour the dressing over the salad and toss to combine. Serve.

SNACKS & SIDES

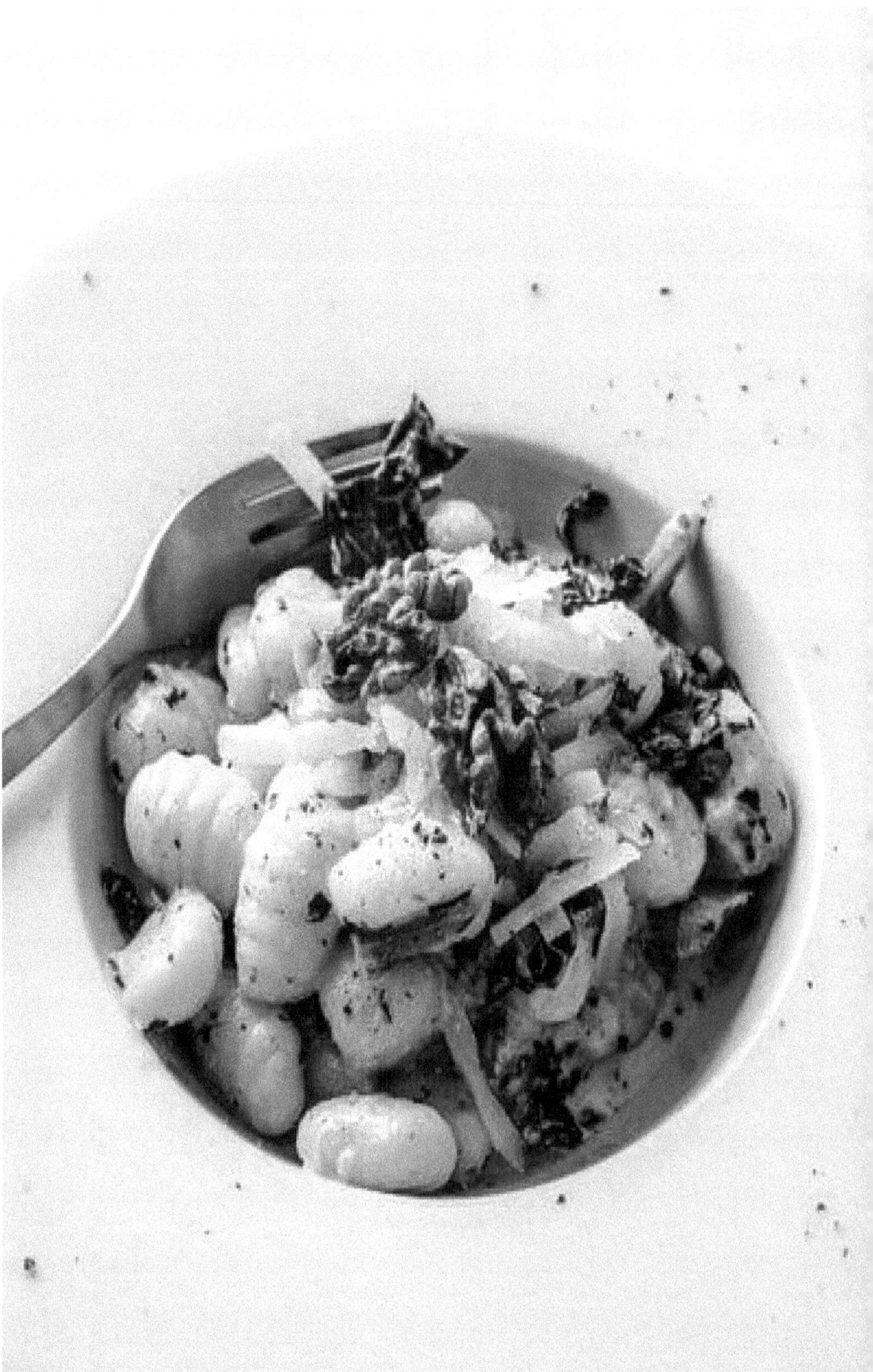

Citrus-Parsley Mushrooms

4 Servings

Preparation time: 15 minutes

Ingredients

- 3 tbsps plant butter
- 3 tbsps fresh lime juice
- 2 garlic cloves, crushed
- 1 tsp dried marjoram
- ½ tsp ground fennel seed
- Salt and black pepper to taste
- 8 oz white mushrooms, stemmed
- 1 tbsp minced fresh parsley

Directions

- Mix the butter, lime juice, garlic, marjoram, fennel seed, salt, and pepper in a bowl.

- Stir in mushrooms and parsley to coat. Marinate covered in the fridge for at least 2 hours.

- Stir to serve.

Mustard Mac & Cheese

4 Servings

Preparation time: 35 minutes

Ingredients

- 8 oz elbow macaroni
- 2 tbsps olive oil
- ½ tsp dry mustard powder
- 2 cups almond milk
- 2 cups plant-based cheddar, grated
- Salt and black pepper to taste
- ¼ cup flour
- 2 tbsps parsley, chopped

Directions

- Cook elbow macaroni in boiling water for 8-10 minutes until al dente. Drain.

- Heat olive oil in a skillet over medium heat.

- Place flour, mustard powder, salt, and pepper and stir for about 3-5 minutes.

- Gradually pour in almond milk while stirring constantly with a spatula for another 5 minutes until the mixture is smooth.

- Turn off the heat and mix in cheddar cheese.

- When the cheese is melted, fold in macaroni and toss to coat. Sprinkle with parsley to serve.

Grilled Vegetables with Romesco Dip

8 Servings

Preparation time: 35 minutes

Ingredients

- 2 (12-oz) jar roasted peppers, drained
- 1 cup toasted almonds
- 2 garlic clove, minced
- 2 tbsps red wine vinegar
- 2 tsps crushed red chili flakes
- 4 slices toasted bread, chopped
- 1 tsp sweet paprika
- 2 tbsps tomato paste
- 1 cup olive oil + 2 tbsps for brushing
- Salt and black pepper to taste
- 2 green bell peppers, julienned
- 2 yellow bell peppers, julienned
- 2 bunch of asparagus, trimmed

Directions

- In a food processor, place roasted peppers, almonds, garlic, vinegar, toasted bread, paprika, and tomato paste;

- pulse, pouring slowly ½ cup of olive oil until the desired consistency is reached.

- Season with salt and black pepper and set aside.

- Heat a grill pan over medium heat.

- Toss the vegetables in the remaining olive oil, season with salt and pepper, and cook in the pan for 3-5 minutes per side.

- Serve with the dip.

Berries, Nuts & Cream Bowl

6 Servings

Preparation time: 30 minutes

Ingredients

- 5 tbsps flaxseed powder
- 1 cup dairy-free dark chocolate
- 1 cup plant butter
- 2 tsps vanilla extract
- 2 cups fresh blueberries
- 4 tbsps lemon juice
- 2 cups coconut cream
- 4 oz walnuts, chopped
- ½ cup roasted coconut chips

Directions

- Preheat oven to 320 F.

- Grease a springform pan with cooking spray and line with parchment paper.

- In a bowl, mix the flaxseed powder with 2/3 cup water and allow thickening for 5 minutes.

- Break the chocolate and butter into a bowl and melt in the microwave for 1-2 minutes.

- Share the vegan "flax egg" into two bowls; whisk 1 pinch of salt into one portion and then 1 teaspoon of vanilla into the other.

- Pour the chocolate mixture into the vanilla mixture and combine well.

- Fold into the other vegan "flax egg" mixture.

- Pour the batter into the springform pan and bake for 15-20 minutes.

- When ready, slice the cake into squares and share it into serving bowls. Set aside.

- Pour blueberries, lemon juice, and the remaining vanilla into a bowl.

- Break blueberries and allow sitting for a few minutes.

- Whip the coconut cream with a whisk until a soft peak forms.

- Spoon the cream on the cakes, top with the blueberry mixture, and sprinkle with walnuts and coconut flakes. Serve.

Simple Vegetable Broth

8 Servings

Preparation time: 45 minutes

Ingredients

- 6 tbsps olive oil
- 4 onions, quartered
- 4 carrots, chopped
- 2 cups celeriac, chopped
- 4 garlic cloves, unpeeled and crushed
- 12 cups water
- 4 tsps soy sauce
- ⅓ cup chopped fresh cilantro
- 2 bay leafs
- Salt to taste
- 1 tsp black peppercorns

Directions

- Warm the oil in a pot over medium heat. Place in onions, carrots, celeriac, and garlic.

- Cook for 5 minutes until softened. Pour in water, soy sauce, cilantro, bay leaf, and peppercorns.

- Bring to a boil, lower the heat and simmer uncovered for 30 minutes.

- Let cool for a few minutes, then pour over a strainer into a pot.

- Divide between glass mason jars and allow cooling completely.

- Seal and store in the fridge for up to 5 days or 1 month in the freezer.

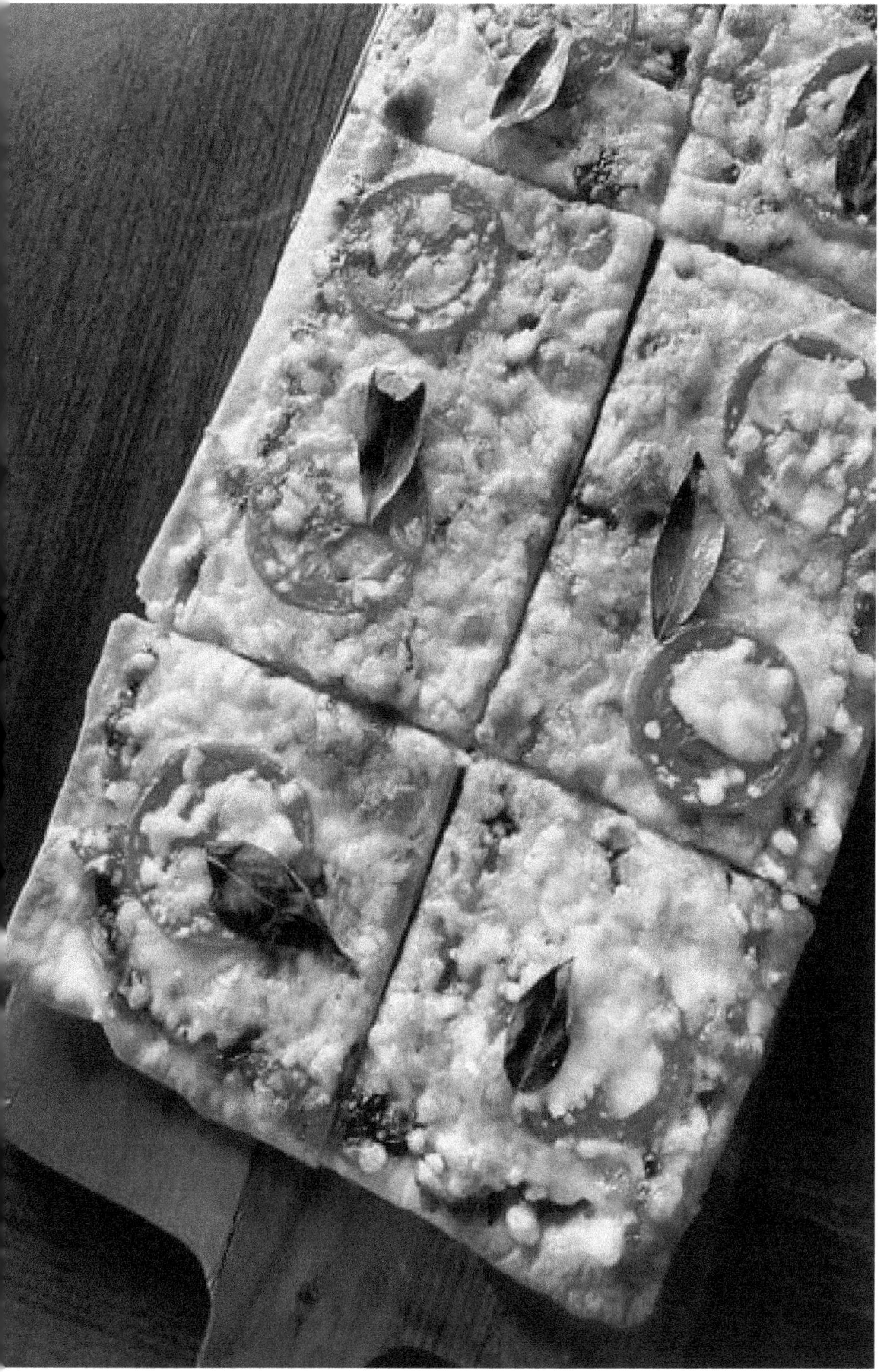

Parsley Veggie Broth

8 Servings

Preparation time: 1 hour 25 minutes

Ingredients

- 2 onions, sliced
- 2 parsnips, chopped
- 2 celery stalk, chopped
- 2 potatoes, unpeeled and chopped
- 6 garlic cloves, minced
- 4 tbsps olive oil
- Salt and black pepper to taste
- 12 cups water
- ⅓ cup chopped fresh parsley

Directions

- Preheat oven to 425 F.

- Grease a baking dish with cooking spray. Put in the onion, parsnip, celery, potato, and garlic and spread them in a single layer.

- Sprinkle with oil, salt, and pepper. Roast the veggies for 30 minutes, turning once by half.

- Let cool for 10 minutes.

- Transfer the vegetables to a pot over medium heat. Add in water, parsley, and salt.

- Bring to a boil, lower the heat and simmer uncovered for 45 minutes until the broth has reduced slightly.

- Let cool for a few minutes, then pour over a strainer into a pot.

- Divide between glass mason jars and allow cooling completely.

- Seal and store in the fridge for up to 5 days or 1 month in the freezer.

Plant-Based Cashew Cheese

8 Servings

Preparation time: 10 minutes

Ingredients

- 2 cups raw cashew nuts
- 4 tbsps freshly squeezed lemon juice
- 4 tablespoons nutritional yeast
- ½ tsp garlic powder
- Salt and black pepper to taste
- ½ cup water or as needed

Directions

- In a blender, process the cashew nuts, lemon juice, nutritional yeast, garlic powder, salt, black pepper, and water until smooth.

- Adjust the taste with more lemon juice, salt, and black pepper as desired and blend again.

- Pour the mixture into an airtight container and use it as the recipe desires.

SOUPS & SALADS

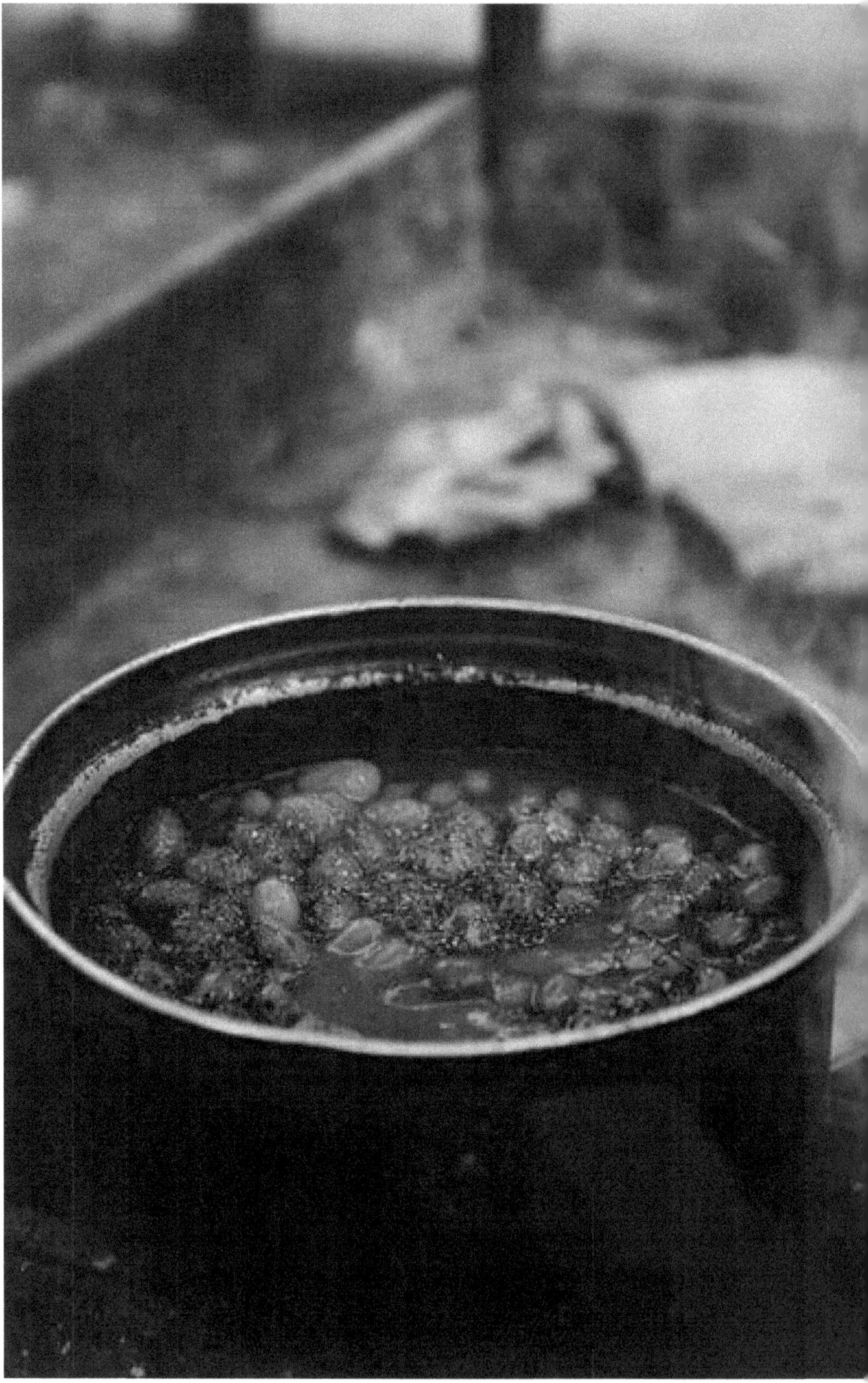

Basil Coconut Soup

6 Servings

Preparation Time: 15 minutes

Ingredients

- 2 tbsps Coconut oil
- 1 cup Green bell peppers, sliced
- 1 (13.5-oz) can Coconut milk
- Juice of ½ Lime
- 2 tbsps chopped Basil
- 1 tbsp chopped Cilantro
- 4 Lime wedges
- 1 ½ cups Vegetable broth
- 2 Garlic cloves, minced
- 1 Onion, chopped
- 1 tbsp minced fresh ginger

Directions

- Heat the coconut oil in a pot over medium heat.
- Add in onion, garlic, and ginger and sauté for 3 minutes.
- Add in bell peppers and broth. Bring to a boil, then lower the heat and simmer.
- Stir in coconut milk, lime juice, and chopped cilantro. Simmer for 5 minutes.
- Serve garnished with basil and lime.

Green Onion Corn & Bean Soup

6 Servings

Preparation Time: 55 minutes

Ingredients

- 2 tbsps Olive oil
- 1 (14.5-oz) can diced Tomatoes
- 1 (15.5-oz) can Pinto beans
- 4 cups Vegetable broth
- 2 cups Corn kernels
- 1 tsp fresh Lemon juice
- Salt and Black pepper to taste
- 2 stalks Green onions, chopped
- Tabasco sauce for garnish
- 1 red Onion, chopped
- 1 red Bell pepper, chopped
- 1 Carrot, chopped
- 2 Garlic cloves, minced
- 1 tsp ground Cumin
- 1 tsp dried Oregano

Directions

- Warm the oil in a pot over medium heat.

- Add in onion, bell pepper, carrot, and garlic. Sauté for 5 minutes.

- Add in cumin, oregano, tomatoes, beans, salt, pepper, and broth.

- Bring to a boil, then lower the heat and simmer for 15 minutes.

- In a food processor, transfer ⅓ of the soup and blend until smooth.

- Return to the pot and stir in the corn. Cook for 10 minutes.

- Drizzle with lemon juice before serving and garnish with green onions and hot sauce to serve.

Celery Butternut Squash Soup

8 Servings

Preparation Time: 30 minutes

Ingredients

- 2 tbsps Olive oil
- 1 Potato, peeled and chopped
- 1 lb Butternut squash, chopped
- 6 cups Vegetable broth
- Salt to taste
- 2 tbsps fresh Orange juice
- 1 Onion, chopped
- 1 Celery stalk, chopped
- ½ tsp ground Allspice

Directions

- Warm the oil in a pot over medium heat.

- Add in onion and celery and sauté for 5 minutes until tender.

- Add in allspice, potato, squash, broth, and salt. Cook for 20 minutes.

- Stir in orange juice. Using an immersion blender, blend the soup until purée.

- Return to the pot and heat. Serve immediately.

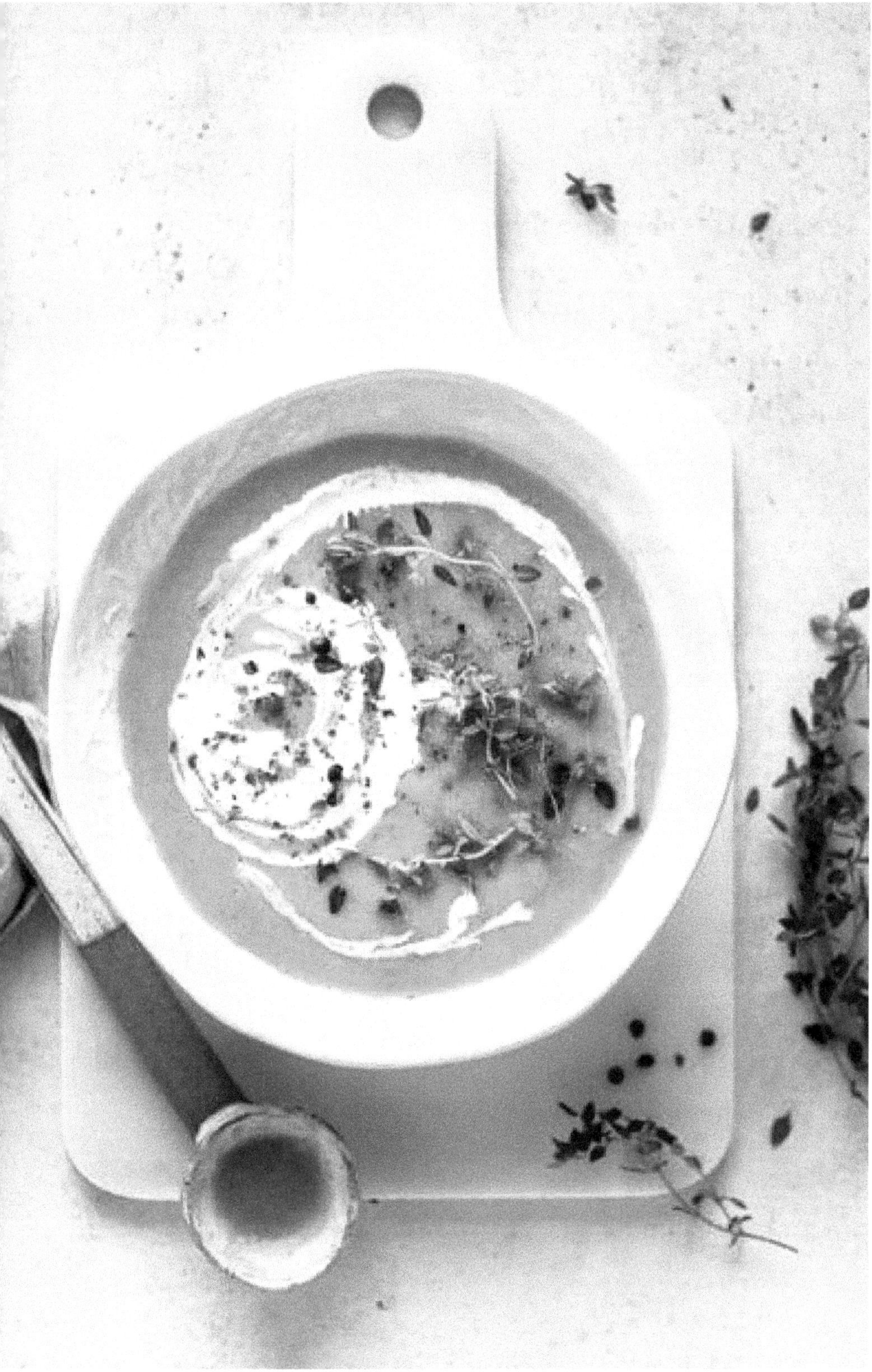

Coconut & Tofu Soup

6 Servings

Preparation Time: 30 minutes

Ingredients

- 1 tbsp Canola oil
- 1 tbsp Pure date sugar
- 1 tsp Chili paste
- 2 cups light Vegetable broth
- 8 oz extra-firm Tofu, chopped
- 2 (13.5-oz) cans Coconut milk
- 1 tbsp fresh Lime juice
- 3 tbsps chopped fresh Cilantro
- 1 Onion, chopped
- 2 tbsps minced fresh Ginger
- 2 tbsps Soy sauce
- 1 cup Shiitake mushrooms, sliced

Directions

- Warm the oil in a pot over medium heat.

- Add in onion and ginger and sauté for 3 minutes until softened.

- Add in soy sauce, mushrooms, sugar, and chili paste. Stir in broth.

- Bring to a boil, then lower the heat and simmer for 15 minutes.

- Strain the liquid and discard solids.

- Return the broth to the pot. Stir in tofu, coconut milk, and lime juice.

- Cook for 5 minutes. Garnish with cilantro and serve.

Ginger Squash Soup

6 Servings

Preparation Time: 30 minutes

Ingredients

- 1/3 cup toasted Pumpkin seeds
- 1 Celery stalk, chopped
- 4 cups Vegetable broth
- 1 Acorn squash, peeled, chopped
- 1 tbsp Soy sauce
- ¼ tsp ground Allspice
- Salt and Black pepper to taste
- 1 cup plain unsweetened Soy milk
- 1 tbsp chopped Ginger paste
- 1 tbsp Canola oil
- 1 Onion, chopped

Directions

- Warm the oil in a pot over medium heat.

- Add in onion and celery and sauté for 5 minutes until tender.

- Add in broth and squash, bring to a boil. Lower the heat and simmer for 20 minutes.

- Stir in soy sauce, ginger paste, allspice, salt, and pepper.

- Transfer to a food processor and blend the soup until smooth.

- Return to the pot. Mix in soy milk and cook until hot. Serve garnished with pumpkin seeds.

Bean & Farro Salad

4 Servings

Preparation Time: 20 minutes

Ingredients

- 1 (14-oz) can Black beans
- 2 Scallions, chopped
- 4 large Whole-grain tortillas
- 2 tsps Olive oil
- 1 tbsp Oregano
- 1 tsp Cayenne pepper
- 4 cups Watercress and arugula mix
- ¾ cup cooked Faro
- ¼ cup chopped Avocado
- ¼ cup mango Salsa
- 1 cup Corn kernels
- ¼ cup fresh Cilantro, chopped
- Zest and juice of 1 Lime
- 3 tsps Chili powder
- Sea salt and Black pepper to taste
- 1 ½ cups Cherry tomatoes, halved
- 1 red Bell pepper, chopped

Directions

- Mix black beans, corn, cilantro, lime juice, lime zest, chili powder, salt, pepper, cherry tomatoes, bell peppers, and scallions in a bowl. Set aside.

- Brush the tortillas with olive oil and season with salt, pepper, oregano, and cayenne pepper. Slice into 8 pieces. Line with parchment paper a baking sheet.

- Arrange tortilla pieces and bake for 3-5 minutes until browned.

- On a serving platter, put the watercress and arugula mix, top with faro, bean mixture, avocado, and sprinkle with mango salsa all over to serve.

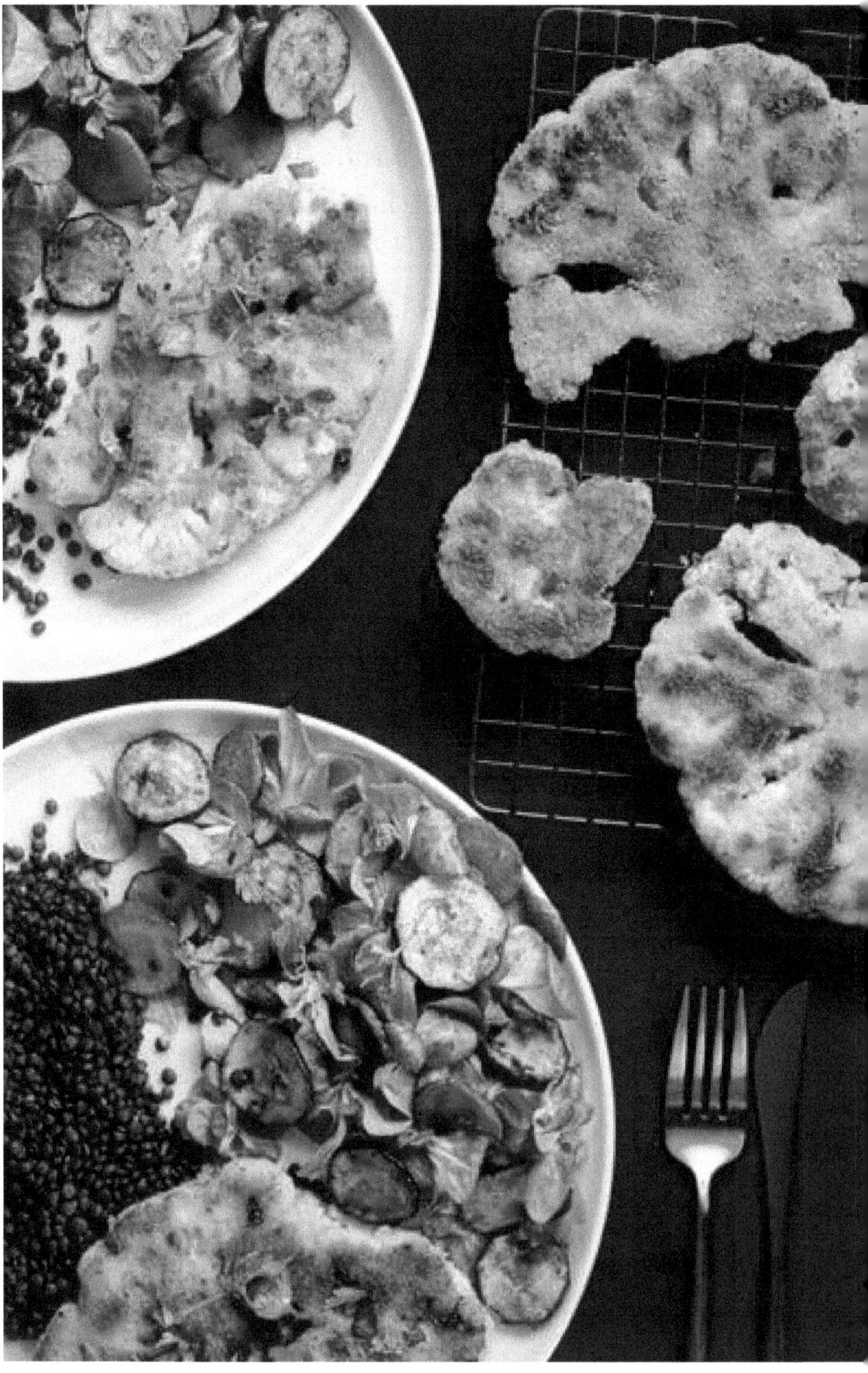

Orange & Kale Salad

6 Servings

Preparation Time: 10 minutes

Ingredients

- 2 tbsps Dijon mustard
- 2 tbsps minced fresh Parsley
- 1 tbsp minced green Onions
- 4 cups fresh Kale, chopped
- 1 Orange, peeled and segmented
- ½ red Onion, sliced paper-thin
- 2 tbsps Olive oil
- ¼ cup fresh Orange juice
- 1 tsp Agave nectar

Directions

- In a food processor, place the mustard, oil, orange juice, agave nectar, salt, pepper, parsley, and green onions. Blend until smooth. Set aside.

- In a bowl, combine the kale, orange, and onion.

- Pour over the dressing and toss to coat. Serve.

African Zucchini Salad

4 Servings

Preparation Time: 20 minutes

Ingredients

- 1 Lemon, half zested and juiced, half cut into wedges
- ½ tsp ground Ginger
- ¼ tsp Turmeric
- ¼ tsp ground Nutmeg
- A pinch of Salt
- 2 tbsps Capers
- 1 tbsp chopped Green olives
- 1 Garlic clove, pressed
- 2 tbsps Fresh mint, finely chopped
- 2 cups Spinach, chopped
- 1 tsp Olive oil 1 zucchini, chopped
- ½ tsp ground Cumin

Directions

- Heat the olive oil in a skillet over medium heat.

- Place the zucchini and sauté for 10 minutes.

- Stir in cumin, ginger, turmeric, nutmeg, and salt.

- Pour in lemon zest, lemon juice, capers, garlic, and mint, cook for 2 minutes more.

- Divide the spinach between serving plates and top with the zucchini mixture.

- Garnish with lemon wedges and olives.

DINNER

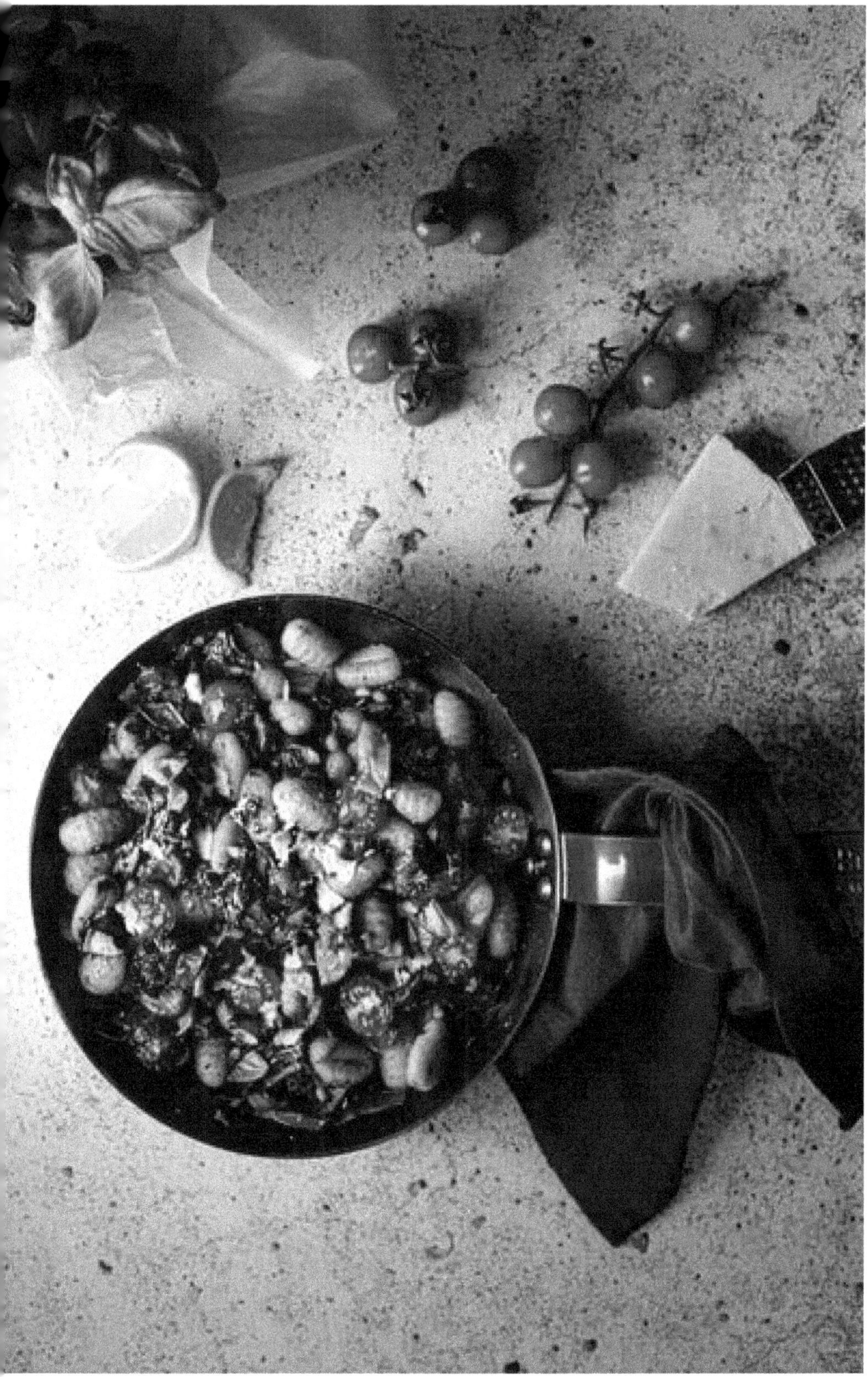

Dilly Potatoes

8 Servings

Preparation time: 35 minutes

Ingredients

- 3 lbs baby red potatoes, halved
- 4 tbsps plant butter
- 6 garlic cloves, minced
- 2 tbsps minced fresh dill
- Sea salt to taste

Directions

- Preheat oven to 430 F.

- Line with parchment paper a baking sheet.

- Mix in the potatoes, butter, garlic, dill, and salt and spread evenly.

- Bake for 30 minutes until golden brown. Serve.

Parsley Faro & Bean Casserole

12 Servings

Preparation time: 50 minutes

Ingredients

- 5 cups water
- 2 cups faro
- 6 tbsps olive oil
- 2 medium yellow onions, chopped
- 2 medium red bell peppers, chopped
- 4 garlic cloves, minced
- 6 cups chopped Swiss chard
- Salt and black pepper to taste
- 2 (15.5-oz) can Great Northern beans
- 2 cups cherry tomatoes, quartered
- 4 tbsps fresh lemon juice
- ½ cup nutritional yeast
- 4 tbsps minced fresh dill weed
- 4 tbsps minced fresh parsley
- 1 cup dry breadcrumbs

Directions

- Boil salted water in a pot over high heat.

- Place in faro, lower the heat and simmer for 30 minutes. Set aside.

- Preheat oven to 360 F.

- Heat the oil in a skillet over medium heat.

- Add in onion and bell pepper and sauté for 5 minutes.

- Stir in garlic, Swiss chard, salt, and pepper.

- Cook for 5 minutes until the chard wilts.

- Remove to the faro pot. Put in beans, tomatoes, lemon juice, yeast, dill weed, and parsley; stir.

- Transfer into a greased baking pan and scatter breadcrumbs over.

- Bake for 10-15 minutes. Serve immediately.

Sicilian Spaghetti Squash

8 Servings

Preparation time: 50 minutes

Ingredients

- 2(4-pound) spaghetti squashes, halved and seeded
- 6 tbsps olive oil
- 2 onions, chopped
- 4 cups chopped artichoke hearts
- 1 cup pitted and sliced green olives
- 2 cups halved cherry tomatoes
- 6 garlic cloves, minced
- 3 tsps Italian seasoning
- Sea salt and black pepper to taste
- Pine nuts
- Plant-based Parmesan cheese
- Red pepper flakes

Directions

- Preheat oven to 390 F.

- Line with parchment paper a baking sheet.

- Rub each squash half with some oil on all sides. Arrange on the sheet cut-sides down and bake for 40-45 minutes until tender. Let cool.

- Meanwhile, heat the olive oil in a skillet over medium heat.

- Place in onion, garlic, and artichoke and cook for 5 minutes.

- Add in olives and tomatoes and cook for another 3-5 minutes. Set aside.

- Take out the squash flesh, using a fork, and separate into strands.

- Transfer to the veggie skillet. Season with Italian seasoning, salt, and pepper; toss to combine.

- Share into bowls and serve garnished with pine nuts, Parmesan cheese, and pepper flakes.

Sesame Tempeh Sauté

8 Servings

Preparation time: 50 minutes

Ingredients

- 8 oz tempeh
- Salt and black pepper to taste
- 2 tsps cornstarch
- 3 cups cauliflower florets
- 2 tbsps canola oil
- 3 tbsps soy sauce
- 2 tbsps water
- 1 tbsp Mirin wine
- ½ tsp crushed red pepper
- 2 tsps toasted sesame oil
- 1 medium red bell pepper, sliced
- 8 oz white mushrooms, sliced
- 2 garlic cloves, minced
- 3 tbsps minced green onions
- 1 tsp grated fresh ginger

Directions and Total Time: 50 minutes

- Combine the soy sauce, water, Mirin wine, red pepper, and sesame oil in a bowl.

- Boil water in a pot and place in tempeh. Simmer for 30 minutes.

- Drain and let cool. Chop tempeh into cubes.

- Transfer to a bowl and sprinkle with salt, pepper, and cornstarch. Set aside.

- Steam the cauliflower for 5 minutes; reserve. Heat the canola oil in a skillet over medium heat.

- Place in tempeh and fry for 5 minutes. Remove to a plate.

- Add bell pepper, mushrooms, garlic, green onions, and ginger to the same skillet and sauté for 5 minutes.

- Stir in cauliflower and tempeh and stir-fry for 1 minute.

- Pour in the Mirin wine mixture and stir to coat. Serve warm.

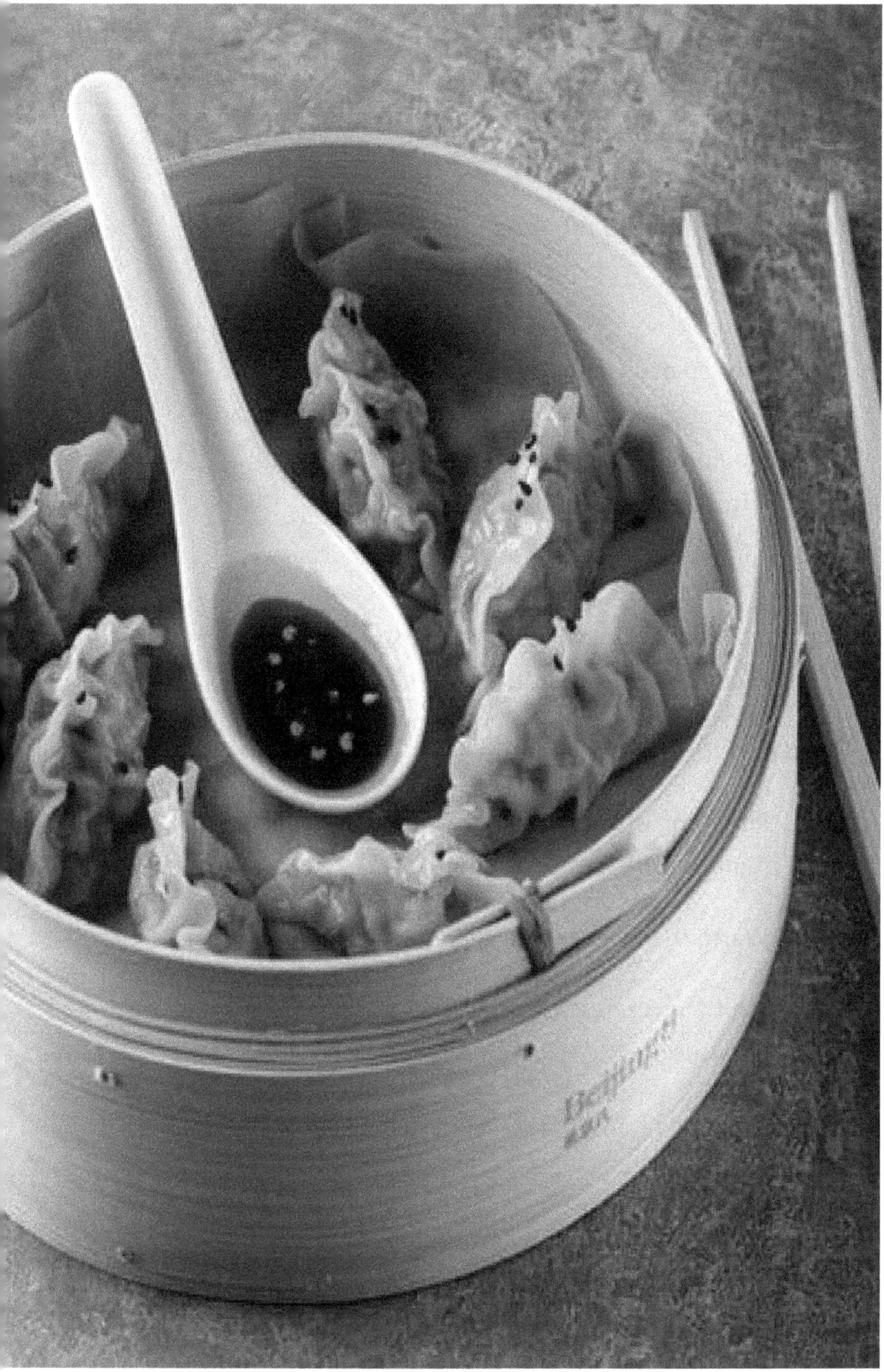

Bell Pepper & Spinach with Walnuts

8 Servings

Preparation time: 15 minutes

Ingredients

- 4 lbs spinach, chopped
- 6 tbsps olive oil
- 2 onions, chopped
- 4 red bell peppers, cut into strips
- 4 garlic cloves, minced
- ½ tsp red pepper flakes
- Sea salt and black pepper to taste
- ½ cup toasted walnuts for garnish

Directions

- Place the spinach in a steamer basket and cook for 5 minutes until tender. Set aside.

- Warm the olive oil in a skillet over medium heat.

- Add in onion, garlic, and bell peppers and sauté for 5 minutes.

- Turn the heat off and mix in spinach, pepper flakes, salt, and pepper.

- Serve topped with walnuts.

Creamy Bell Pepper Goulash

8 Servings

Preparation time: 50 minutes

Ingredients

- 4 tbsps olive oil
- 2 onions, chopped
- 4 garlic cloves, minced
- 2 potatoes, chopped
- 2 lbs bell peppers, chopped
- 2 tbsps tomato paste
- 1 cup dry white wine
- 3 tbsps sweet paprika
- 2 tsps caraway seeds
- 3 cups sauerkraut, drained
- 3 cups vegetable broth
- 1 cup vegan sour cream

Directions

- Heat the oil in a pot over medium heat.

- Place in onion, garlic, bell peppers, and potato and sauté for 8-10 minutes.

- Mix in tomato paste, wine, paprika, caraway seeds, sauerkraut, and broth.

- Bring to a boil, then lower the heat and sprinkle with salt and pepper.

- Simmer for 30 minutes.

- Whisk 1 cup of cooking liquid with sour cream in a bowl.

- Pour into the pot and adjust the seasonings if needed. Serve hot.

Thyme Black Bean Loaf with Artichokes

12 Servings

Preparation time: 45 minutes

Ingredients

- 2 potatoes, chopped
- 2 (10-oz) package artichoke hearts
- ½ cup olive oil
- 2 onions, chopped
- 2 (15.5-oz) can black beans
- ½ cup vegetable broth
- 4 tbsps tahini
- 3 tbsps soy sauce
- 3 tbsps fresh lemon juice
- 2 cups whole-wheat flour
- 1 cup nutritional yeast
- 2 tsps dried thyme
- Salt and black pepper to taste
- 1 cup chopped sun-dried tomatoes
- ½ cup minced fresh parsley

Directions

- Preheat oven to 360 F.

- Place the potatoes and artichokes in hot water and steam for 15 minutes.

- Drain and set aside. Cut 2 artichoke hearts and set them aside.

- Heat the oil in a skillet.

- Place onion and sauté for 3 minutes. Add in potatoes and artichokes.

- Remove to a blender and add beans, broth, tahini, soy sauce, and lemon juice. Pulse until smooth.

- In a bowl, combine the flour, yeast, thyme, salt, and pepper.

- Pour the potato mixture into the flour mixture. Add in sun-dried tomatoes, parsley, and reserved artichokes.

- Toss to coat. Shape the mixture into a loaf and place in a greased loaf pan to bake for 40 minutes until golden brown.

- Leave to cool for 15 minutes. Slice and serve.

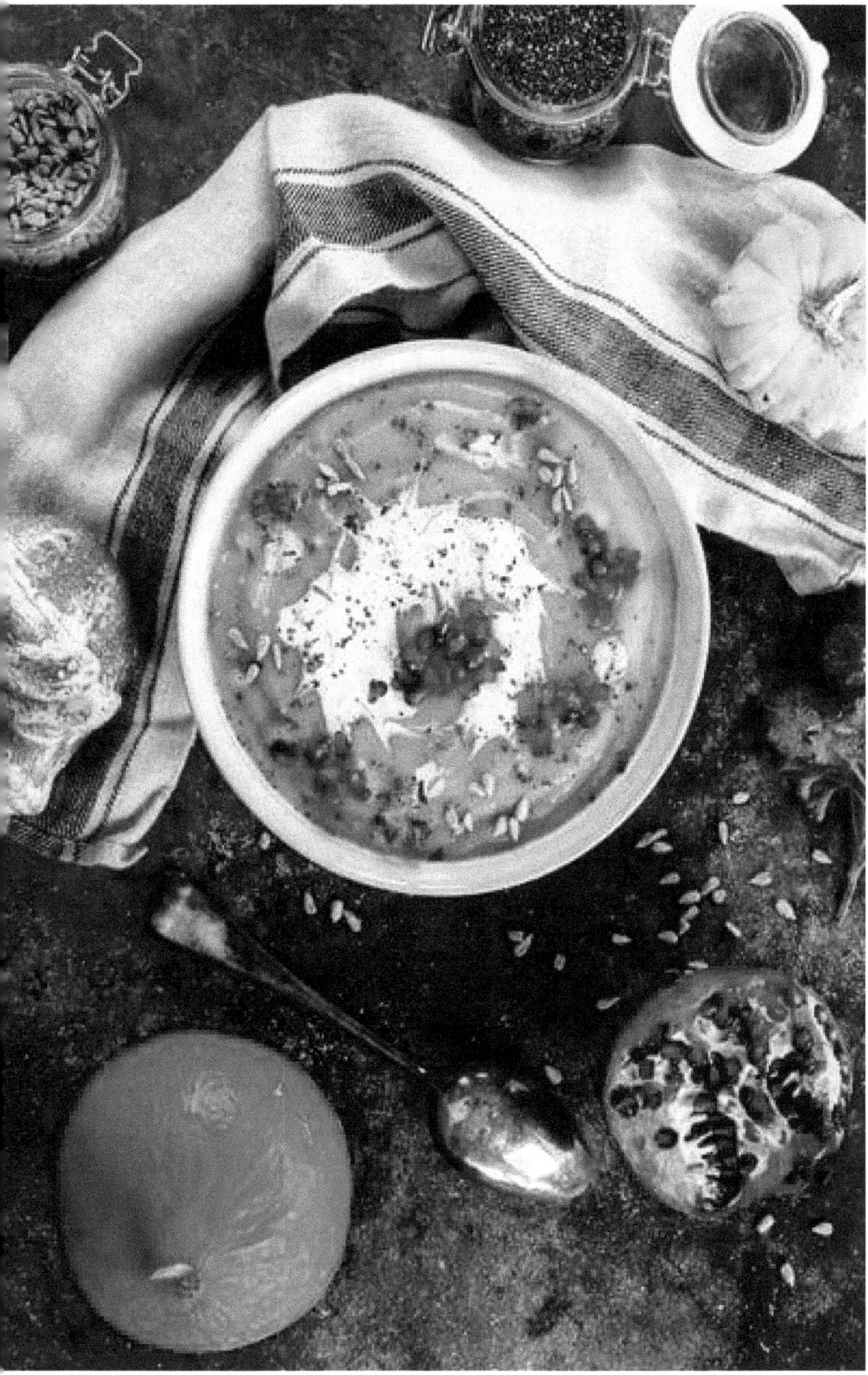

Pomegranate Bell Peppers & Eggplants

8 Servings

Preparation time: 40 minutes

Ingredients

- 1 cup olive oil
- 2 onions, chopped
- 6 eggplants, cut into chunks
- 2 red peppers, chopped
- 2 yellow bell peppers, chopped
- 4 garlic cloves, minced
- 2 hot chili, seeded and minced
- 4 tbsps pomegranate molasses
- 1 cup orange juice
- 4 tsps pure date sugar
- 2 ripe peaches, chopped
- 1 cup finely chopped fresh cilantro

Directions

- Heat the oil in a skillet over medium heat.

- Place the onion and sauté for 5 minutes. Add in eggplants, bell peppers, garlic, and chili.

- Cook for 10 minutes.

- Stir in pomegranate molasses, orange juice, sugar, salt, and pepper.

- Bring to a boil, then lower the heat and simmer for 20 minutes until the liquid reduces.

- Top with peach and cilantro and serve right away.

DESSERTS

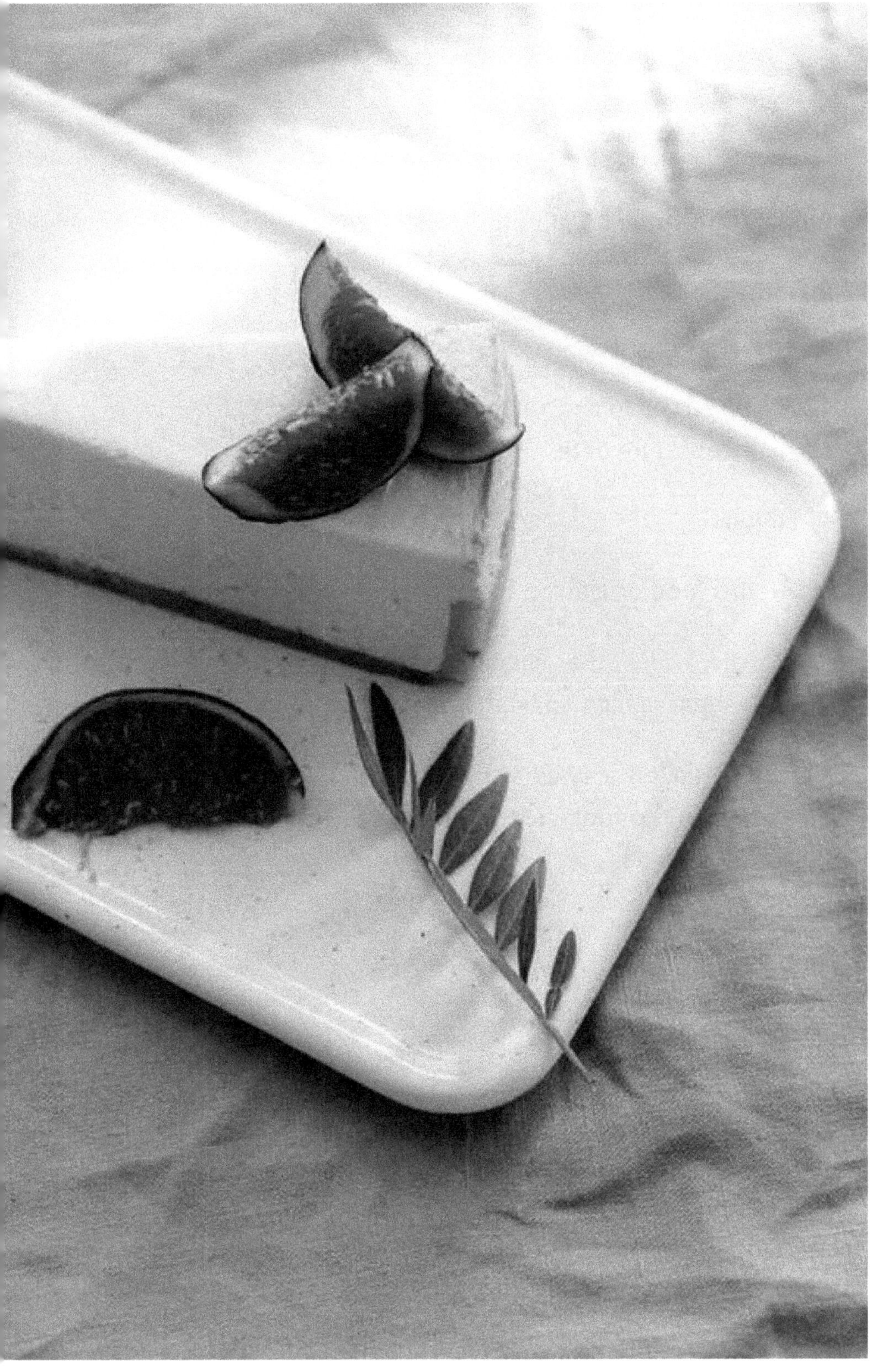

Mango Chocolate Fudge

3 Servings

Preparation Time: 15 minutes

Ingredients

- 1 mango
- ¾ cup vegan chocolate chips
- 4 cups pure date sugar

Directions

- In a food processor, blend the mango until smooth.

- Microwave the chocolate until melted. Add in the pureed mango and date sugar and stir to combine.

- Spread on a lined with waxed paper baking pan and chill in the fridge for 2 hours. Once chilled, take out the fudge and lay on a cutting board.

- Discard the waxed paper. Slice into small pieces and serve.

Coconut & Chocolate Macaroons

4 Servings

Preparation Time: 25 minutes

Ingredients

- 1 cup shredded coconut
- 2 tbsps cocoa powder
- 1 tbsp vanilla extract
- ⅔ cup coconut milk
- ¼ cup maple syrup
- A pinch of salt

Directions

- Preheat oven to 360 F.

- In a pot, place the shredded coconut, cocoa powder, vanilla extract, coconut milk, maple syrup, and salt.

- Cook until firm dough is formed. Shape balls out of the mixture. Arrange the balls on a lined with parchment paper baking sheet.

- Bake for 15 minutes. Allow cooling before serving.

Sicilian Papaya Sorbet

4 Servings

Preparation Time: 5 minutes

Ingredients

- 8 cups papaya chunks
- 2 limes, juiced and zested
- ½ cup pure date sugar

Directions

- Blend the papaya, lime juice, and sugar in a food processor until smooth.

- Transfer the mixture to a glass dish. Freeze for 2 hours.

- Take out from the freezer and scrape the top ice layer with a fork. Back to the freezer for 1 hour.

- Repeat the process a few more times until all the ice is scraped up.

- Serve frozen garnished with lime zest strips.

Hazelnut Topped Coconut Caramelized Bananas

4 Servings

Preparation Time: 15 minutes

Ingredients

- 2 bananas, peeled, halved crosswise and then lengthwise
- 2 tbsps coconut oil
- 2 tbsps coconut sugar
- 2 tbsps spiced apple cider
- Chopped hazelnuts for topping

Directions

- In a skillet over medium heat, melt the coconut oil. Place in bananas, cook for 2 minutes. Turn them, cook for another 2 minutes.

- Pour the sugar and cider around the bananas, cook for 2-3 minutes, until thickens and caramelize.

- Serve into bowls topped with remaining liquid and hazelnuts.

Apple & Cashew Quiche

6 Servings

Preparation Time: 55 minutes

Ingredients

- 5 apples, peeled and cut into slices
- ½ cup pure maple syrup
- 1 tbsp fresh orange juice
- 1 tsp ground cinnamon
- ½ cup whole-grain flour
- ½ cup old-fashioned oats
- ½ cup finely chopped cashew
- ⅔ cup pure date sugar
- ½ cup plant butter, softened

Directions

- Preheat oven to 360 F. Place apples in a greased baking pan. Stir in maple syrup and orange juice.

- Sprinkle with ½ tsp of cinnamon. In a bowl, combine the flour, oats, cashew, sugar, and remaining cinnamon.

- Blend in the butter until the mixture crumbs.

- Pour over the apples and bake for 45 minutes.

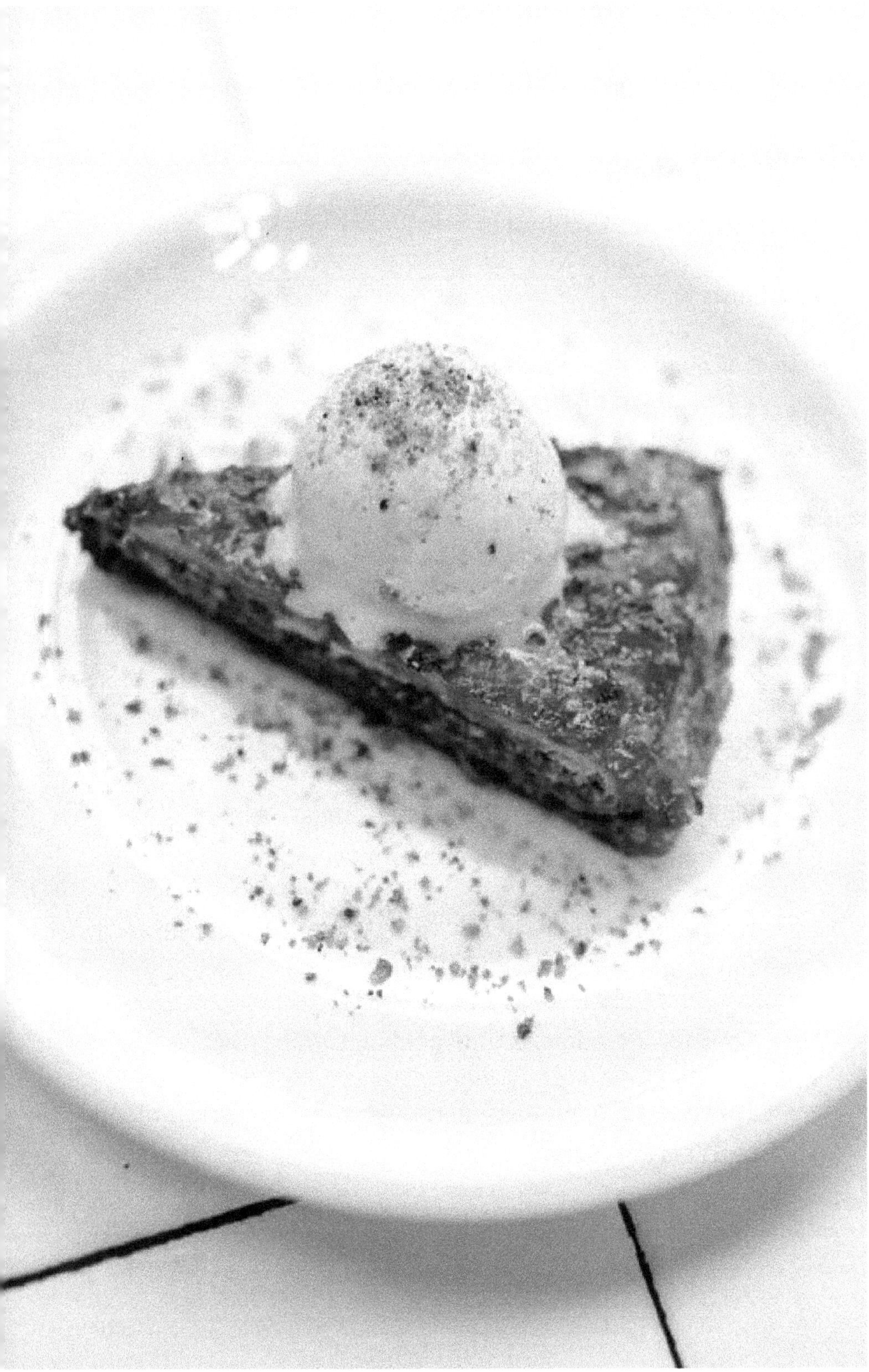

Tofu & Almond Pancakes

10Servings

Preparation Time: 15 minutes

Ingredients

- 1 ⅓ cups almond milk
- 1 cup almond flour
- ⅓ cup firm tofu, crumbled
- 3 tbsps plant butter, melted
- 2 tbsps pure date sugar
- 1 ½ tsps pure vanilla extract
- ½ tsp baking powder
- ⅛ tsp salt

Directions

- Blitz almond milk, tofu, butter, sugar, vanilla, baking powder, and salt in a blender until smooth.

- Heat a pan and coat with oil. Scoop a ladle of batter at the center and spread all over.

- Cook for 3-4 minutes until golden, turning once.

- Transfer to a plate and repeat the process until no batter is left. Serve.

Almond Berry Cream

4 Servings

Preparation Time: 15 minutes

Ingredients

- 3 (15-oz) cans almond milk
- 3 tbsps maple syrup
- ½ tsp almond extract
- 1 cup blueberries
- 1 cup raspberries
- 1 cup strawberries, sliced

Directions

- Place almond milk in the fridge overnight. Open the can and reserve the liquid.

- In a bowl, mix almond solids, maple syrup, and almond extract.

- Share berries into 4 bowls. Serve topped with almond cream.

Lightning Source UK Ltd.
Milton Keynes UK
UKHW020656140521
383710UK00001B/69

9 781802 854084

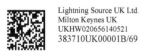

.